MW01152352

9/1/09

Karla dear,

This book is for you!

— Deanna

Alzheimer's: Days Gone By

For those caring for their loved ones

By: Deanna Lueckenotte, BA,
LNFA, LBSW, CALM

authorHOUSE®

AuthorHouse™
1663 Liberty Drive, Suite 200
Bloomington, IN 47403
www.authorhouse.com
Phone: 1-800-839-8640

© *2009 Deanna Lueckenotte, LBSW, CALM, LNFA. All rights reserved.*

No part of this book may be reproduced, stored in a retrieval system, or transmitted by any means without the written permission of the author.

First published by AuthorHouse 6/17/2009

ISBN: 978-1-4389-6749-3 (e)
ISBN: 978-1-4389-6748-6 (sc)

Printed in the United States of America
Bloomington, Indiana

This book is printed on acid-free paper.

Contents

Preface vii
Acknowledgments ix
Chapter 1 - Taking Care Of Yourself 1
Chapter 2 - Behaviors 13
Chapter 3 - Communication-Is it possible? 19
Chapter 4 - Daily Living 29
Chapter 5 - Lifestyle Enhancement Programming 41
Chapter 6 - Overview of Dementia 49
Chapter 7 - Inside the human brain 59
Chapter 8 - Research 65
Chapter 9 - Resources 71
Chapter 10 - Forget Me Knots 77
Chapter 11 - Hope For Holidays 87
Chapter 12 - Home Safety 93
Chapter 13 - Light in the Tunnel Stories 101

PREFACE

"Days gone by" with Alzheimer's can seem like an eternity for caregivers faced with the challenges of taking care of someone with the disease. Alzheimer's, at this time, still remains progressive and irreversible with no cure for the person inflicted with it.

My sincere goal of this book is to help caregivers find a little light in this darkened tunnel that you must travel. This is not a quick fix guide. This book is a compass to help during the times when you are feeling lost. Keep it close to you and refer to it often.

When caring for someone with Alzheimer's learn to let go of your reality and enter their reality wherever they may be. As you go through this journey you will continue to learn and experiment with the concepts presented to you. This book is geared to help all types of caregivers no matter the setting. Alzheimer's is all around us, some of us may not realize how much because we have not been educated in the signs of Alzheimer's. You can come in contact with someone facing this disease while you are eating out or shopping!

I am writing this book to meet the needs of you who may, at some time in your life, be faced with someone in their "days gone by!" Keep looking for the light in the tunnel and remember that some days the light will be brighter than others!

My prayers remain with you and with everyone in "days gone by."

ACKNOWLEDGMENTS

This book is dedicated to my mom who was also my best friend. Her journey with cancer led me into a tunnel that I thought had no light. Through the years, mom you keep reminding me from up above, how to find even the smallest light in the tunnel for others as well as myself. I love you and thank you for all your blessings and insight that your life and death bestowed upon me.

I also want to thank my family and friends for being so patient with me during the time it took to write this book. All of you mean so much to me. Also, to Jo Blaylock with Elder Options of Texas for reading, rereading and helping critique this book. Dr. Angie Hochhalter PHD, who is an assistant professor in the department of medicine at Scott & White Memorial hospital and Texas A&M Health Science Center, Temple ,Texas. Know that your section on research in this book will touch so many lives and that you are an inspiration to many. Continue your research on Alzheimer's.

Your personal journeys have made you wonderful advocates for care-givers facing Alzheimer's. Thank you for taking the time to help me dot my i's and cross my t's throughout my own journey with this book. Jo and Dr. Angie Hochhalter know that you have been my light and inspiration at the times I felt discouraged about my writing abilities.

Special thanks to Robert Falcon who is a licensed funeral director and embalmer in the State of Texas and has over 20 years experience in the funeral service industry. He has been recognized by national and local funeral consumers groups for his continued efforts in inform-ing families about their consumer rights, making meaningful funeral arrangements, and providing affordable services. Robert is a native of Austin, TX, where he established two very successful funeral homes. Robert thanks for teaching me to shop even for death and helping me educate others on prearrangements!

Mrs. Dottie Bishop, my third grade teacher, thank you for inspiring me so many years ago in regards to writing. Per our conservation so long ago I promised to acknowledge you when I wrote my first book!

To Bryan, my partner in life: Thanks for helping me believe in my own abilities and my passion for Alzheimer's! No one would be reading this book today if it was not for you. Your constant wisdom of saying to me over and over "When are you going to stop talking about writing it and actually do it?" helped me overcome my fears inside of myself.

To the special people that allowed me to put their "light in the tunnel" stories into this book. It made it so much more than could have been imagined. You know who you are and you also know that your stories are helping others through their journeys. You each are a blessing and I hope you continue to find "light in your tunnel."

NOTES

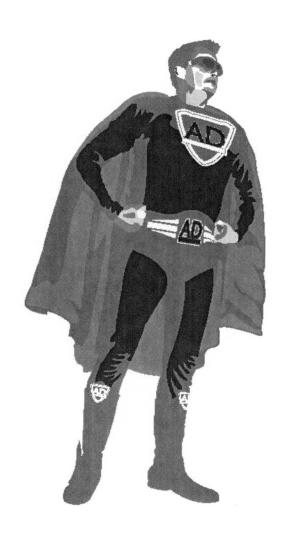

Chapter One

Taking Care Of Yourself

Taking Care Of Yourself

Dementia caregivers are very special people. The demands seem to require super human abilities at times. If you take better care of yourself, you will be better prepared to provide care for your loved one, family members, and anyone else who may need your help.

Some of the unique demands put on you:
- The person with Alzheimer's may not recognize you from day to day
- They may strike out physically
- They are often unable to give back
- You may not receive a thank you.
- They get worse no matter how good your care is.
- The routine they need may become monotonous for the caregiver.
- The times that they have an alert moment can leave you with a feeling of false hope which keeps you on an emotional roller coaster to say the least!

Some of the special skills a caregiver needs include:
- Willingness to learn and change due to the inability of your loved one to understand, compromise or change for you
- Patience
- Good listening skills
- Sense of humor
- Flexibility
- High self-esteem
- Self-direction
- Positive attitude
- More desire to give than receive
- Open minded
- Sense of self responsibility and creativity

This list is not all inclusive and you can add to your own list at any time.

It is okay to realize that you are a "super person!" With all of these super human abilities stress will play a big part in your life.

Stress is characterized by the body's own specific response to the varying demands that are placed upon it. Many times stress is referred to in a negative light; however, stress can help to keep a person alert and motivated allowing the person to accomplish more than they would have otherwise. The stress test below will give you an idea of where you are in regards to managing your stress.

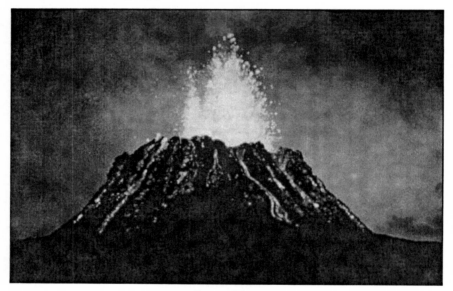

Stress Test

1. I can't get enough sleep.

2. I have conflicts with other family members.

3. I feel anxious.

4. I feel like I have no time for myself.

5. I worry that I am not doing a good job as a caregiver.

6. I feel depressed, trapped or resentful.

Scoring system: Add your points up per question by this scale.

Never=0
Sometimes=1
Usually=2
Almost Always=3

0-7 You are managing fairly well.

8-12 It's time to consider some additional support.

13+ You are already experiencing a degree of burnout.

The goal in treating stress is not to eliminate stress but to learn how to manage it and use it to your advantage. You will see that a manageable amount of stress motivates you to excel in your performance and unmanageable levels of stress can suffocate and overwhelm you.

Find a stress reliever that works for you:
- A five minute breath of fresh air may help you to be a better caregiver for the rest of the day.
- It is okay to ask for help.
- Go outside and drink a cup of tea.
- Walk your dog.
- Do something for you!
- Practice deep breathing techniques.
- Try a silent scream or scream into a pillow.
- Duck into a quiet spot and give a silent scream.
- Cool off by counting to 10.
- Step back from the situation, take a break and try again.

Ways to manage your stress:
- Take care of your own health.
- Talk to someone you trust about your problems and feelings.
- Look on the bright side.
- Share the work with your family.
- Be organized and plan ahead.
- Take responsibility.
- Find what causes stress in your life and notice your reaction to the stress.
- Identify areas of your life you can change to eliminate or

reduce negative reactions to stress.
- Build up your emotional ability to handle stress.
- Exercise to increase your physical capacity to deal with stress.
- Teach yourself to control your physical reactions to stress.

Warning signs of frustration:
- Knot in the throat
- Shortness of breath
- Desire to strike out
- Compulsive eating
- Chest pains
- Stomach cramps
- Headaches
- Increased smoking
- Excessive alcohol consumption
- Lack of patience.

If you start to feel out of control ask for help. You may have super human abilities but some times your cloak does not protect you. Have fun, enjoy life, and find those lights in the tunnel with your loved one!!

Ways to take care of yourself include:
- Learn to be gentle with yourself.
- Find a hermit spot and use it daily.
- Remind yourself that you are an enabler and not a magician.
- Learn to say "I choose" rather than "I should", "I ought to", or "I can't".
- Keep in mind if you never say "no" what will your "yes" be worth?
- Take time to laugh and play.
- Find support systems that can help you through the dark times in the tunnel.

Let's take a laughter test to see how much humor and laughter are in your life.

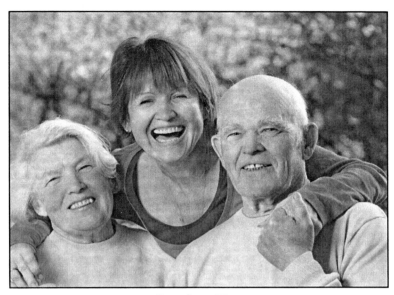

Laughter Test

Read each of the following ten statements and write a number from 1-5 representing the phrase below which best describes your feelings about each statement.

1 for strongly agree; 2 for agree; 3 for sometimes; 4 for disagree; and 5 for strongly disagree

<u>Score</u>

1. I feel I have a good sense of humor.
2. I enjoy laughing and do so easily.
3. I feel comfortable laughing by myself whether in private or public.
4. I enjoy laughing at home with family and do so easily.
5. I enjoy laughing at work and do so easily.
6. I make a point of sharing the funny stories or jokes I hear.
7. I like making other people laugh and consider myself fairly good at it.
8. People tell me I have a good sense of humor.

9. I often try to turn tense moments around by using humor.
10. I seek out people and things that make me laugh.

<u>Total</u>   _____

1-50	*You are not laughing enough.*
1-39	*Read a humorous book.*
1-29	*You're laughing just enough to get by.*
1-19	*You're laughing a lot.*

It is very difficult on any family that is in the situation of dealing with a loved one with Alzheimer's. Family members go through more stages of adjustment when dealing with Alzheimer's than they do if they were to lose a loved one due to death.

There are 6 stages of adjustment when you lose someone to death and 10 stages for families faced with a family member with Alzheimer's. All the feelings, fears and frustrations you have are expected and it is part of your adjustment to facing the fact that your loved one has Alzheimer's. In a sense you lose your loved one twice...first to Alzheimer's and then to death!

TEN STAGES OF FAMILY ADJUSTMENT

Stages   What families may say.

Stages	What families may say.
Shock	Why me? This can't be true!
Denial	My wife is not like others with Alzheimer's; My mom will learn bad habits from the others with Alzheimer's.
Fear and anxiety	Will I have this burden for the rest of my life; Will I get this disease?
Guilt/anger and blow up cycle	Sometimes I wish she would die; When she asked the same question again I yelled at her.
Social withdrawl	I don't want people to see mom like this; I must be strong and not ask for help.

Depression and grief	There is no hope; Nothing is fun anymore; I am all alone.
Letting go	It is hard for me, but I can accept help; It is okay to have a good time.
Hope	I can see a light at the end of the tunnel.
Truth	It is okay for others to take care of my wife.
Loving with no strings	I will always have a place in my heart for my loved one but I can form new relationships.

As the caregiver you may experience irritability, sleepless nights, health problems, exhaustion and lack of concentration during your adjustment to caregiving. Depression is another issue you may face while taking care of your loved one. Many caregivers have symptoms or have been diagnosed with depression. If you see signs of depression contact your doctor and ask for help. It is okay to ask for help. Illness associated with caregiving includes but are not limited to cancer, diabetes, and heart disease.

As a caregiver you may be also faced with becoming the "parent" in your relationship with your loved one. It is difficult for the child or spouse to transition and adjust to this new role in their loved one's life. Sibling issues of other family members not wanting to make decisions, taking little to no responsibility, and refusing to transition into the parental role can add more stress, guilt, denial and depression to you the caregiver, who chooses to become the "parent."

Financial burdens will increase due to the need for care giving assistance at home or the difficult decision to place your loved one in a long term care facility. Unavoidable decisions can add financial stress to other stressors you are facing. Another financial stressor is due to little public funding available to help caregivers with expenses. Research and educate yourself on all your options in regards to your financial situation.

Caregivers with positive attitudes suffer less caregiver burden while caregivers that have more of a pessimistic attitude will experience higher levels of burden. If you keep a more upbeat attitude you will experience less caregiver burden. When the caregiver experiences more behavioral issues from their loved one with Alzheimer's this can also increase chances of experiencing caregiver burden.

Caregivers continue their own lives which include responsibilities of everyday living. For example: Working another job outside of taking care of your loved one, other personal relationships, parenting your own children and everyday domestic and financial duties! Imagine living life with all these stressors for 5 to 20 years!!!

Overall, with all the stressors (also known as "caregiver burden") and adjustments that the caregiver is faced with it is no surprise why caregiver's develop "super human abilities." As the caregiver remind yourself that even superhero's take breaks periodically, blow off steam at times or bring in sidekicks to help. Learn to take care of yourself so you can continue to take care of the one's that must rely on you!

NOTES

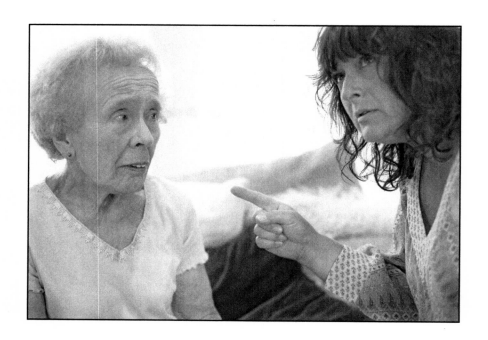

Chapter Two

Behaviors

Behaviors

How many of you have heard that behaviors just happen in Alzheimer's and it is part of the disease process and there is nothing you can do to change it????? After finishing this chapter you will have a different understanding of behaviors in dementia type including Alzheimer's. Regarding behaviors and Alzheimer's you need to think of yourself as a private investigator. Learn to enjoy looking for ways to alleviate their behaviors. Look at it as finding the piece of the puzzle that fits for them! All behavior has meaning. Don't give up finding the meanings behind the behaviors in your loved ones. Please remember that the only time failure occurs is if you stop trying!

There are some causes of behaviors which include but are not limited to over stimulation (loud noises, too crowded), unfamiliar surroundings, current surroundings offering too many options, hunger, <u>PAIN</u> and un-comfortable due to being too hot, cold, clothing too tight, or positioning. They may become overwhelmed due to a higher functioning activity or communication with loved one which may cause frustration.

Three steps in helping to deal with challenging behaviors are to iden-tify and examine the behavior (ask: what, when, why, how and where?). Explore different solutions and try different responses if needed. The main concept is that each behavior may require a different answer each time your loved one exhibits the behavior. That is what makes behaviors in your loved one faced with Alzheimer's so challenging.

It is a good idea to keep a log of behaviors that are exhibited along with the who, what, when, where type philosophy. This will allow you to find out triggers of your loved ones behaviors. Granted you may not see it at first but overtime you will see the patterns.

You may see that your loved one becomes more agitated after a visit from someone. You can monitor the visits and you may discover that the visitor is unknowingly frustrating your loved one by asking them reality type questions. Or maybe the visitor is placing demands on your loved one who can no longer do the task. For example: The visitor may be asking your loved one to tell them how to make their famous chili. You as the caregiver could educate your visitor to the fact that they do not remember the recipe but that you have written down. Plan a time for the visitor to come over and cook the chili and have your loved one help as much as possible within their failure free limits. Everyone can enjoy a good meal together also.

Below are definitions and a chart with interventions for behaviors that you as the caregiver may see throughout their disease process.

- **Exit seekers** have a specific goal to wandering.
- **Explorers** like to see and touch things.
- **Followers** like to follow others.
- **Pacers** have the need to move due to excess energy.
- **Verbal repetitive behaviors** include repeating the same question, story or statement over and over again.
- **Physical repetitive behaviors** include rummaging, banging, moving tongue, rubbing hands, and tapping feet.
- **Aggressive behaviors** include angry outbursts, hitting, throwing things, biting and yelling or screaming.
- **Paranoia** is an unreasonable suspiciousness and puts unrealistic blame on another.
- **Hallucinations** are feeling, hearing, tasting, seeing, or smelling things that are not there.
- **Catastrophic event** is an extreme emotional response that is out of proportion compared to the actual event. Some examples include: striking out, anger, rapid mood changes, increased restlessness, and uncontrollable crying.
- **Sun Downing** occurs more in the afternoon. They may become more disoriented which may cause more frustration or overwhelming feelings which in turn leads to more behaviors

  •

Behaviors and Interventions

Repetitive behaviors (Verbal & Physical)	Wandering(Exit Seekers, Followers, Explorers, and Pacers	Aggression	Paranoia and hallucinations	Catastrophic event
Remember they are not doing this to annoy	Monitor their whereabouts	Watch for signs of frustration	Do not argue with them	REMAIN CALM
Give them an object to hold	Walk or pace with them/ include in activity	Try to sooth them and talk with them about their emotion	Offer reassurance that they are safe	Maintain safety of self and loved one
Respond to the emotion	Offer food and drink	Assess the danger level	Stay calm and treat fear as real	Let expression of feelings occur
Try to redirect	Try to redirect	Stay calm	Try to redirect	Try to redirect
Involve in a activity/snack	Ensure the environment is safe	Redirect them to an activity	Try to include in a activity	Asses what caused event and avoid in future
Always assess PAIN	Always assess PAIN	Always assess PAIN	Always assess PAIN	Always assess PAIN

Please remember that there are many different interventions. This table is a guideline. Think outside of this chart and explore what works for you and your loved one. PAIN can cause more agitation and behaviors in anyone whether they have a dementia or not. For example: If you had a headache, toothache, hunger, thirst or did not sleep well the night before how would you react if I approached you and said "Come on so we can get you in the shower!"

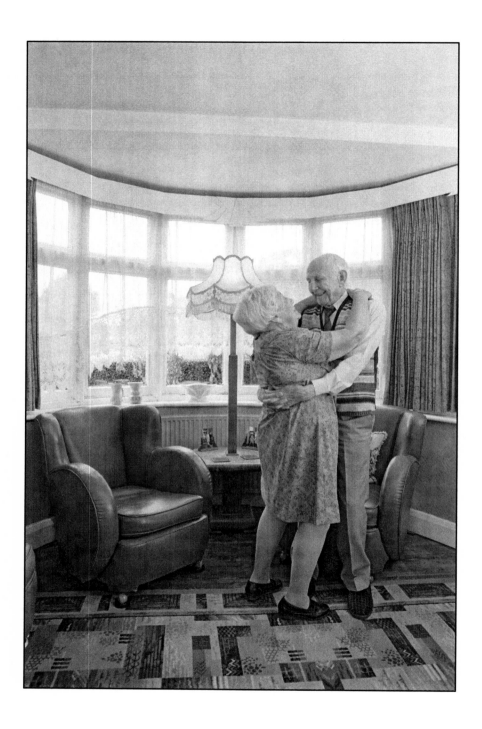

Chapter Three

Communication-Is it possible?

Types of Communication

There are two types of communication which include verbal and nonverbal. Verbal is the use of meaningful words, nonsense or made up words, singing, sounds and shouts. Nonverbal is the use of body language. Nonverbal communication is done with our eyes, touch, facial expressions, gestures, hand movements, body posture and position.

There are 3 components to communicating which include body language, vocal tone, and content. Think about these 3 components and what percentage each part plays in communicating. You may be surprised at the percentages listed below.

- Body language   55%
- Vocal Tone   38%
- Content   7%

As you can see the nonverbal (body language) is a very important aspect when communicating with others. Keep this in mind when communicating with your loved one. Just because they may have trouble with the content does not mean that they can't pick up on what you are saying. Your loved one can pick up on frustration, fear, happiness, sadness, anger and other body language.

There are nonverbal strategies for effective communication. Maintain a calm pleasant approach. The person with dementia will mirror your mood. If you act rushed or tense the dementia person may react by becoming more anxious or agitated. Approach the person from the front to minimize the startle effect. Always establish eye contact. Speak at eye level whenever this can be done. Point or demonstrate what you are trying to get across.

There are also verbal strategies for effective communication. Use a calm gentle voice. Use short simple sentences. Speak slowly. Call the person by name and introduce yourself if necessary. Answer a frequently asked question like it was the first time they have asked it. Eliminate distracting noises. Give one instruction at a time. Do not overwhelm them. Remember you are speaking to an adult. Allow enough time for the person to respond and repeat yourself if necessary. Use words that are familiar to them.

There are also things not to say which include but are not limited to trying to argue with them, talking louder when they do not understand you, using a demanding tone and asking questions that rely on the use of memory if experiencing a disoriented moment. You should treat them the way you would want to be treated under the same circumstances. Basically, try to put yourself in their shoes.

There are general communication tips to help alleviate the barrier you are facing with your loved one. Be a good listener. Encourage nonverbal types of communication and be patient and supportive. Show interest in what they are saying and do not criticize. Focus on feelings and not the facts and offer comfort and reassurance. Limit distractions, offer a guess when they can not find the word and give them time to express their thoughts. Use cue cards to help with communication barriers. Do not make fun of their lack of abilities or tease them at any time. Once again…Do Not Argue. I know I have said that before but I can not emphasize the importance of not arguing with your loved one.

Communication with someone with Alzheimer's can be a difficult task. Keep in mind when communicating to enter their reality instead of bringing them into yours. Below are some examples of ways to communicate with your loved one. There are many ways to communicate other than the ones I have listed. Hopefully, you will take these ideas and come up with what works best for you in the situation that you are currently in. It is a trial and error process and what works today may not work tomorrow. Use your own skills and implement your own ideas. The main concept is to limit reality orientation to little or none depending on where your loved one is in their own reality. For example: If your loved one states "I know my husband is dead but I do not remember where he is buried." This person could handle some reality orientation. On the other hand if the person states "I need to be home to cook dinner for my husband." (Her husband has been dead for 10 years) This would not be a good time to use reality orientation with someone. Reminiscing, validation, good cop/bad cop or redirection may work better during times of disorientation. We will discuss therapy techniques in more detail a little later. These are techniques to use to help you and your loved one with communication and behavioral issues. It is not lying to your loved one but techniques used to help you through your journey. Below are a few examples of ways to communicate with your loved one.

1. My husband is waiting for me to cook dinner. I have to leave now!

Your husband called and said to eat dinner without him because he is running late. (Keep in mind you may be their husband but in their mind you are not that person!) You do not want to go into an involved detailed story. Keep it simple. Also do not say things like "He stopped off at the local bar." or "He had a flat tire." Statements like these may even upset your loved one even more. You also do not want to tell them that their husband has been dead for 10 years even if it is the truth. Research and find out why her husband was late in the past.

2. My children will be home soon. I need to go home!

Ask more questions about their children. How many children do you have? Tell me a cute story about one of your children. You try to get their mind off of finding the exit.

3. Where is my wife? I can't find her.

Ask questions about his wife. Same as the other questions we have gone over. Think about it and come up with different ways to redirect your loved one. Validation or reminiscing may also work well.

Alzheimer's disease damages parts of the brain that control communication so each person may experience communication impairments that include word finding-trouble which is finding the right words. Memory loss may cause the person to repeat themselves over and over again. They may have difficulty following conversations. They may have automatic speech which is a phrase they have said over and over again like "thank you." Curse words may be used more frequently due to the disease process. They may be able to still read but not comprehend what they are reading.

Communicating with the hearing impaired can add to your already difficult situation. In the elderly as we know our hearing may fail us so it is important to discuss some strategies to incorporate with the other communication tips you just read about. If they have a hearing aid, encourage them to wear it and check the batteries often. If they did not have a hearing aid before the disease process started it will be a challenge to keep the hearing aid in their ear. They may feel that it does not belong or it may confuse and scare them because of the ability to hear well. Write things down if needed. Get their attention by saying their name and gently touching your loved one's shoulder. Stand directly in front of the person when speaking to them. Speak slowly and clearly and use a lower tone of voice. Use nonverbal communication such as gesturing or pointing. Approach them from the front.

Communicating with the visually impaired can also be a barrier due to deterioration that takes place as we age. Here are a few tips to use when facing this barrier. Use large print when communicating. Avoid startling them. Tell them what you are going to do before you start your care. Avoid loud noises or sudden movements. Identify yourself as you approach. If they have eye glasses, encourage them to wear them. Keep them clean and check the prescription routinely. Laminate a group of pictures that represent what you are trying to communicate. For example: Laminate a picture of a bathroom, a plate of food, toothbrush and toothpaste,etc. Another technique that will help you in regards to communicating is to talk with your loved one about their history in regards to childhood, young adult and early married life. Find out about special, traumatic, and funny events that occurred in their life. If they are unable to communicate their life history then talk with other family members that can help fill in the blanks. Take the information you gather and put it into a journal so you have access to it throughout the disease process. This journal will help you find lights in the tunnel during your journey. It will help you fill in the blanks when they can no longer communicate details to you.

When you listen there are two types of information you need to get. Factual information which are the facts and emotional information which allows you to see inside the other person. Ask open ended questions allowing the person to express their feelings. Below is an exercise on open ended questions to help you learn more ways to gather emotional information. Keep in mind that open ended questions require more than a yes or no response.

Exercise on open ended question

Which questions below are open ended?

1. Did you feel bad when she said that to you?
2. Why did you say that?
3. What was it like hearing that from someone you care for?
4. Were you afraid?
5. Was it difficult?
6. What did you mean to say?
7. Are you angry?
8. How do you feel when you become frustrated?

The questions that you can answer yes or no to mean that it is not an open ended question and you will not get much information from these types of questions. Once they progress further into the disease process you may need to use less open ended questions due to their abilities.

When you listen to others you assume you know what the speaker is saying because of your own past experiences. Only about 10% of us listen properly and poor listening habits create communication breakdowns. Listening is a skill. It is an active process. It is focused. It takes concentration and effort and it is the key to communication. Growing up I loved to talk (I still do!) and my mom would remind me that I was given only one mouth and two ears and so I was meant to listen more than talk!

As already mentioned there are different techniques to use with an Alzheimer's person including reality orientation, validation therapy, good cop/bad cop, reminiscing and redirection. You may be using validation therapy and then 5 minutes later you may be switching over to redirection. You will be kept on your toes and will need to use the tools and tips in listening and communication to make life easier for you.

Reality orientation typically means to bring them into today's reality. My definition of reality orientation is to enter their reality instead. *If they think it is 1940 then in their reality it is 1940. If they think it is 2005 but unsure gently reorient them to the present.* This technique is where the caregiver helps the person regain their awareness of person, place, and time. It can be useful in the early stage if the information reassures your loved one. It can upset the person in middle or later stages if they cannot recall or understand what is told to them.

Validation therapy is a concept in which the emotion is responded to rather than the statement itself. It can help reduce stress and establish a bond. There are things to keep in mind while offering validation which includes entering their reality. Look for feelings behind the words or behaviors that are being exhibited. Be non-judgmental. Empathize with your loved one. Remain calm at all times. Provide reassurance and comfort. Allow your loved one to express feeling including negative ones.

Good cop/bad cop is great to use when you have someone else with you when a behavior occurs. For example if your loved one is angry with you and a visitor is present you can become the "bad cop" while the visitor can become their buddy ("good cop") until the behavioral episode passes. It is important to educate all your visitors on all the different techniques that can be used while visiting.

Redirection is the action of trying to distract your loved one from negative thoughts or actions. Methods of diversion can include offering an activity, food, and task to complete but is not limited to these.

Communication is also a day by day process. What works today may not work tomorrow but may work the next day! Your super human abilities of patience and perseverance will definitely be used during the communication process. Remember the only time failure occurs is if you stop trying!

NOTES

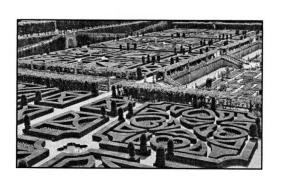

CHAPTER FOUR

DAILY LIVING

Daily Living

Cognitive changes can cause activities of daily living (ADL's include dressing, bathing, toileting, personal hygiene, etc) to become more difficult. Memory loss in the early stage can cause the person to become less independent. They may forget how often they have worn the clothes or the last time they showered or bathed. They may forget how to operate an appliance like a washing machine. They may have trouble dressing themselves appropriately.

During the middle stage they may become increasingly confused which can lead to humiliation or embarrassment regarding needing help with toileting or showering. They may lose the ability to make a decision on what to wear or what sequence to use in dressing. They may feel overwhelmed toward all the clothing in their closet. They may also experience confusion on the need to be dressed or undressed. They may have a fear of falling and have a decreased ability in using a shower or bathtub.

Physical changes can also affect the person's ability to remain independent due to decreased ability to hear or see which makes it more difficult to follow instructions. Balance can become an issue which will make dressing difficult. Loss of motor skills makes activities of daily living more difficult. Poor circulation and illness due to flu or infection may bring about less motivation to take interest in personal hygiene or cooperation regarding hygiene. Depression can also affect independence for them.

There are ways to encourage them to participate in personal care. Avoid arguing! If they resist walk away and try again later. Try to have a distraction free area. Focus on their abilities. Encourage independence. For example: If you are brushing their hair and they are unable to do this any longer then give them a hair brush to hold in their hands. Use good communication techniques. Break down instructions into steps instead of overwhelming them. Take extra time and do not rush. By spending extra time you may stop them from becoming more agitated later on due to becoming overwhelmed. If you rush and if they become agitated it will take you more time to work through the agitation than it would have taken you to take the time with the activities of daily living!

Toileting can become a challenge during the Alzheimer's process. It may become more common for a person with Alzheimer's to have less control over bowel and bladder functions. Some causes of incontinence include stress. Common signs of leakage will occur when coughing, laughing, or sneezing. Drinking coffee, alcohol, or citrus juices can irritate the bladder or cause inadequate hydration. Medical conditions including urinary tract infection (UTI), fecal impaction, enlarged prostate and vaginitis can also cause more challenges in toileting. Medications including anti-histamines, sedatives, diuretics, medications with caffeine like aspirin or Excedrin, and blood pressure medications can also bring about challenges in toileting. They may not recognize the natural urge or forget where the bathroom is located and how to use the facilities.

Tips for toileting include establishing a schedule for reminding them to use the toilet or offering assistance to the toilet. Remove obstacles that may be in the way of the path to the toilet. Also make sure clothing is easy to remove. Provide cues and look for cues. Post a picture of a toilet on the bathroom door. Colored toilet lids may help the toilet stand out. Look for non-verbal cues from them like increased agitation, crossing and uncrossing legs, picking with a belt or zipper of pants, opening or closing of doors, or grabbing their personal area. It is a good idea to monitor incontinence and to look for a pattern so you can get them to the restroom before the typical time of incontinence occurs. This will help alleviate accidents and help with your frustration. Limit fluid intake later in the evening and schedule a bathroom time in the middle of the night. Be supportive by helping them retain a sense of dignity even with the incontinence issue. Having a reassuring attitude will help with feelings of embarrassment. Think about different words that describe "toileting." They may not understand you if you refer to it as the bathroom but if you referred to it as the "john", "outhouse", "the girls closet", "toilet", "head", or "restroom" they might go directly to the toilet! Another reason bathroom may not work is during the disease process they may establish a fear of water and may associate "bath"room to mean shower time. Use your private investigator skills that I mentioned earlier. Put your thinking caps on when it comes to dealing with behaviors during activities of daily living.

Bathing can be the most difficult care activity that a caregiver will face. The person with Alzheimer's may feel they are being threatened during this process and they may scream, hit, or resist. To try to help overcome the unpleasant experience prepare the bathroom in advance. Have everything you need supply wise before bringing them in. Put all the items you need into a personal caddy for them so you are not trying to run around the house finding everything. Also check the temperature of the room and water. None of us like a cold room or a cold bath. Help them feel in control by involving in and instructing them through each step of the process. Include them even if it is holding a washcloth while you bath them. Be gentle because skin can be very sensitive. Avoid scrubbing and pat dry instead of rubbing. Most people do not like water all over their face when taking a bath so please keep that in mind. You can try putting a towel over their face and head area to keep the water away while showering rest of the body and then use a "no rinse" type shampoo if needed. You can also try washing their hair in the kitchen sink. Another option is to take them to have their hair washed and set once a week. This may be an especially good fit for a woman. If they were a bath person instead of a shower person research options available that would allow them to bath in a safe setting. Keep the bathroom as homelike as possible. Distractions and noises should be limited.

Dressing the person with Alzheimer's also presents a challenge. They may not remember how to dress or be overwhelmed by the choices involved in dressing. Dressing and physical appearance is important to everyone's self-esteem. Also keep this in mind while helping your loved one dress and do not rush them. To help the person with dressing try to simplify choices and keep closets free of excess clothing. Choose comfortable and simple clothing. Substitute velcro for buttons, snaps, or zippers that may be too difficult for them to handle. Organize the process for them. Lay out the clothing in the sequence it needs to be put on or hand the clothing to them one article at a time. Use short simple instructions like "put on your shirt" instead of "get dressed." Offer accessories because most people like to "dress up" at times. Limit distractions and be flexible. If they want to wear the same outfit ever day try to get duplicates or a close match. In later stages give them a piece of material they can hold while you are putting their clothing on.

Eating properly is important in staying healthy. Regular intake of food may become a problem for someone with Alzheimer's due to being overwhelmed by too many food choices. They may think they have already eaten or forget to eat at all. Use bright color dishes due to the contrast in the color of the food from the plate which will help increase their food intake. When helping your loved one eat keep in mind these points. Make mealtime comfortable and a calming experience. Consider adaptive equipment to encourage eating independently. Have dentures checked routinely. Offer one food at a time and monitor for choking hazards. Offer finger foods and supplements and encourage independence. Take away all utensils not being used to prevent them from feeling overwhelmed. Pre cut foods and de-bone food items for safety. Do not use individual packets of condiments because they may try to eat them. Do not offer small containers of jelly, cream, or butter because this may overwhelm them. Napkins should be loose instead of wrapped-up. Serve soup in cups so they can drink it easier.

Also keep in mind they may have built in beliefs that they may not be able to voice any longer. For example: During their childhood years they were taught to pray before eating. Also, is there someone at the table wearing a hat? Some people will not eat until all hats have been removed. It may be as simple as needing to set the table before eating. Another detail to watch is the intake of their food. If they start eating the dessert (sugar items) first, or only eating the dessert, it may be time to start putting a little sugar on all the foods. The one taste that typically lingers for someone with Alzheimer's is the sweet taste. Always check with your family doctor first to make sure that adding more sugar to your their diet will not do more harm than good. They may not feel "hunger" like they once did or they may forget completely how to chew and swallow during the last stage of Alzheimer's.

Dental care is also very important because proper care of the teeth and mouth can help prevent digestive problems, eating difficulties, and extensive dental procedures. This activity of daily living can also be a difficult task because they may forget how to brush their teeth and the importance of this task.

Here are some simple procedures to follow in regards to brushing their teeth. Provide short simple instructions. Instead of saying "Brush your teeth" you may need to say "Hold your toothbrush in your hand", "put toothpaste on the brush", and "brush your teeth." Use a technique called mirroring. Hold the toothbrush and show them how to brush their teeth or even put your hand over their hand and gently guide the brush. Check daily to ensure oral care has been done. Brush teeth at least twice a day. Remove and clean dentures every night. Don't forget to brush the gums and roof of mouth. Keep a watch out for signs of discomfort during meal time. This may indicate mouth pain or dentures that do not fit correctly.

Some general tips to follow while assisting with any activity of daily living include working with them as an adult, deserving respect. Encourage independence and pay attention to nonverbal communication. Do not talk to them as though they are not there. Break tasks into steps that match their abilities. Experiment with new approaches and give encouragement, reassurance, and praise. Use short direct simple words and keep instructions simple. Remember that sometimes slowing down is the fastest way to accomplish something!

Other activities of daily living that you as a caregiver may face include inappropriate wearing of shoes. This occurs typically in the middle and late stages. They may begin to take shoes off or walk around with one shoe on and one off. If this happens assess their feet as well as the shoes for physical problems. If no problems it could be the dementia process so try different types of shoes that are washable and discard the other type of shoes so there will be no argument in the future. If they are unable to keep shoes on then try slipper socks with grips.

Another challenge you may face is women resisting to wearing bras. This will typically take place in the middle and late stage. If resistance occurs to wearing a bra assess body areas for physical problems, the bra for comfort and other problems. If still resistant try a sports bra because of softness and stretch. If there is a continued issue with bra wearing you may want to use an undershirt instead for dignity issues as well as comfort. Keep in mind the following question (for women): Do you like to wear a bra from the time you wake up until you go to bed? I would imagine that your answer is not in this lifetime! Why do we expect our loved one to do something we ourselves would not do? Think about it!

Men resisting to shave or be shaved is also a challenge you could face. This may occur in middle to late stage. As the caregiver, assess skin for physical problems and make sure the shaving equipment is working properly. If he is still resistant have another family member shave him. If it continues to be a problem talk to other family members and ask if he had a beard when he was younger. He may think he is 40 years old and if he had a beard during that age why in the world would someone be shaving it off? Attempt every day to shave. If needed allow beard to grow until receptive but keep the beard groomed and clean. An electric razor may also be another option to try.

Disrobing may also occur during the middle and late stage. Here are a few things to help with disrobing challenges. Assess skin for any physical problems and assess clothing for proper fit. If nothing found and behavior continues you may want to invest in elastic waist pants, over the head blouses or dresses or sweat suits because it is harder to disrobe out of this type of clothing. Supportive appliances (dentures, eyeglasses, hearing aids) will begin to be removed by them and at times they will completely stop using them. This increases as the disease process increases. They may lose the ability to understand what the supportive appliance use is. In regards to supportive appliances assess for physical problems as well as the appliance itself. Assess them to see if level of dementia has increased. You can do this. Look in the earlier chapter and think back to where they were and where they are now. Try a different way to help them keep using the supportive device such as elastic straps on eyeglasses. Use appliance during times that will enhance the care given. Supportive appliances should be stored in a safe, clean area when not in use.

In regards to supportive appliances know that if they wore eyeglasses since they were 10 then they will still want their eyeglasses on. If they can not find their own they will wear any that they can find. On the other hand if they never wore glasses until later in life you as the caregiver will have more trouble getting them to wear the appliance. It is a tough battle with appliances and take each day one day at a time regarding eye wear, dentures, walkers, hearing aids and etc.

Stage Specific and Activities of Daily Living

Early (Mild)	Middle (Moderate)	Late (Severe)
Needs help choosing clothing	Needs help putting clothes on in correct order	Needs total assistance in dressing
May need coaxing to bathe	Needs help getting to bath and washing and drying	Needs total assistance in bathing
May need help locating bathroom and reminders	Needs help locating toilet and how to use the appliance	Needs total assistance in toileting
Feeds self with minimal assistance	Needs meal process simplified (finger foods, pre cut foods, condiments put in food and drinks	Meal needs to be very simplified. Will take food off of others plates. Will pour liquids into food. May eat package of condiments. Generally like sweet tasting foods. May need total assistance in feeding

Here are some tips for caring for someone with late-stage Alzheimer's. Eating during the latter stage creates special challenges. Make sure they have comfortable seating. Allow more time for meals. You may need to change their food type. For example: Puree. Encourage self feeding but assist if needed. Maintain a quiet environment. Realize that you may become more frustrated and that it is okay to feel this way.

Skin issues in late stage Alzheimer's also presents challenges. Keep skin dry and clean. Alleviate body pressure and protect bony areas. Watch out for decubitis which are break down of the skin.

Tips for toileting issues in late stage Alzheimer's include limiting liquids before bed. Use adult briefs if necessary. Set a toileting schedule. Monitor bowel movements. Eliminate caffeinated drinks due to being a diuretic.

Ways to reduce risk of infections and pneumonia in late stage include cleaning gums and tongue. Keep an eye on oral hygiene. Keep a log of cuts and abrasions and treat them immediately. By keeping the log you know how long they have had the abrasion and if it has worsened or not. You may think you will remember but with everything going on in your life you may not remember what it looked like a week earlier.

NOTES

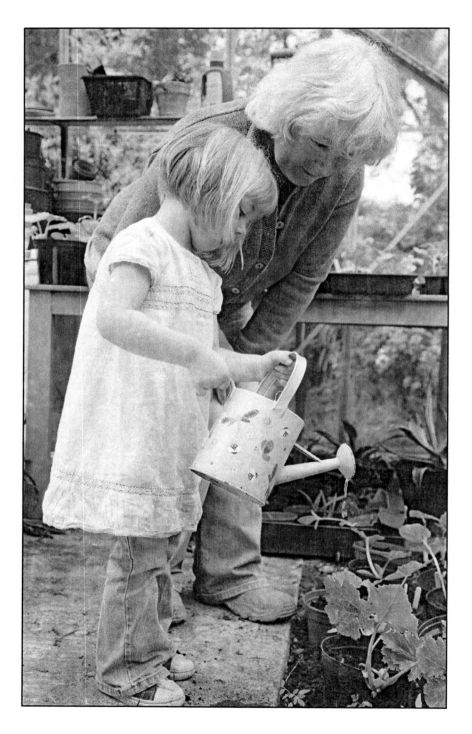

CHAPTER 5

LIFESTYLE ENHANCEMENT PROGRAMMING

LIFESTYLE ENHANCEMENT PROGRAMMING

Lifestyle enhancement programming means exactly what it says. It is a program to enhance the person suffering with Alzheimer's. An activity is anything and everything a person does each day. This includes getting dressed, playing cards, doing chores, dancing, etc. Different forms of activities include but are not limited to personal care activities which are taking care of one's self such as eating, drinking, and dressing. Leisure activities is time spent on hobbies, recreation, or cultural experiences which include singing, dancing, walking, socializing, puzzles, arts, crafts and reminiscing. Productive activities are tasks that make one feel useful and needed like table setting, dusting, sweeping, folding, sorting or clearing tables. Insightful activities include religious services, spiritual reading, singing hymns or praying.

When planning activities with them have a list of hobbies and things they like from their past and present. Assess the activity with their abilities to make sure they will not be overwhelmed or frustrated because the activity that is presented is too hard. Also assess to make sure that the activity you are giving them will not embarrass or belittle. They may not enjoy the hobbies that they have enjoyed for the last 40 years. Activities are a great deal like behaviors. You need to be a private investigator and try different things. Also keep a log of things that they respond well to as well as things they do not respond well to. You set a schedule that works for them. You must remain flexible within your structure because they are always changing their capabilities. Going back to your log will help you keep up with where they are. As they grow in the Alzheimer's process you need a chart to know where they are and where they are going next.

Below is a list of activities that people have come up with for others with Alzheimer's disease. Copy this list and highlight the ones you think they would enjoy and add your own to the list. Assess each activity for their ability to perform each one. Keep in mind that this list is not complete so add to it as you can. Keep an open mind in regards to activities.

- Clipping coupons
- Reminisce about the first day of school
- Give a manicure or pedicure
- String Cheerios to hang outside for the birds to eat/put bird feed out
- Dye Easter eggs
- Pop popcorn
- Put coins into jars(You may need to supervise due to small items)
- Ask simple trivia
- Sew sewing cards
- Make a birthday cake
- Have afternoon tea
- Make a fruit salad
- Toss a ball or balloon
- Look at family pictures
- Make sandwiches
- Sort objects
- Sing songs
- Wash silverware and put away
- Take a walk
- Sort playing cards
- Remember great inventions
- Fold towels
- Arrange flowers in a vase or basket
- Sort socks
- Reminisce
- Dance
- Have a spelling bee
- Wipe off a table
- Fold clothes
- Make fresh lemonade
- Look up names in a phone book
- Sort poker chips
- Read from newspaper or readers digest
- Bake cookies
- Have children, babies, and pets visit

- Listen to relaxing music
- Plant seeds
- Sweep the patio
- Roll yarn into a ball
- Finish Bible quotations
- Sand wood
- Mold with play dough
- Look at magazines
- Straighten underwear drawer
- Put a simple puzzle together
- Rub in hand lotion
- Finish nursery rhymes
- Finish famous sayings
- Cross word puzzles
- Snap beans
- Work in the garden
- Exercise
- Stretch
- Baking
- Seasonal crafts
- Painting
- Drawing
- Have treasure boxes for reminiscing. For example: wedding, soldier, babies, first day of school, etc.
- Put shows/skits together that may interest your loved one. Examples: doll, hat, fashion, car, puppet shows and etc.
- Watch movies/television that your loved one watched years ago. Examples include Shirley Temple, Bonnanza, Leave It To Beaver, Brady Bunch, and etc.
- Go on an outing. For example: Church, Bowling, Train ride, Senior Center Events

During an activity offer support and supervision to them and always be patient. Count to ten, take a deep breath, and find what works for you. Concentrate on the process not the outcome. Be realistic and relaxed. Stress a sense of purpose. Let them know they are needed. Help get the activity started. Be flexible. Assist with difficult parts of the task. Break activities into simple easy to follow steps. Don't criticize or correct.

Substitute an activity for a behavior. For example if they can not keep their hands still maybe it is time to snap some peas. Involve them through conversation. If they do not want to participate try again later. You may also want to try a different activity if they do not respond well.

Lifestyle enhancement programming will benefit them by encouraging independence. It will help them feel useful. It will alleviate some of your frustrations. It also creates positive self expression and feelings. It encourages socialization with others. It is important to be with our peers no matter what age we are. Social engagements help anyone feel connected and establish a sense of belonging. It entertains them. It will provide spiritual guidance as well as intellectual stimulation. It will help improve self-esteem.

NOTES

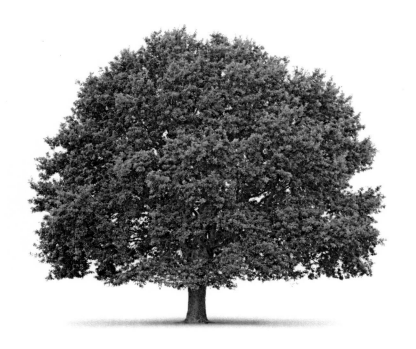

CHAPTER 6

OVERVIEW OF DEMENTIA

Overview of dementia

Today we are faced with 5.5 million people inflicted with this disease right now and the number continues to grow. We are also living longer which will increase the number inflicted. Add the baby boomer generation to this and it will be explosive!

Before you take your journey to find the light in your tunnel you need to know about dementia and memory. Learn a little about the inside of the human brain, the different types of dementia, stages, treatment and research regarding Alzheimer's.

Throughout our busy lives we may have trouble remembering things from time to time. For many people some forgetfulness is a completely normal part of the aging process. Please keep in mind that memory loss can also be a symptom of something more serious than forgetfulness. If the memory loss interferes with daily life it could be the first symptom of Alzheimer's disease. An example of interference in daily life could be a transcriptionist who now can't remember how to transcribe any longer. Another example is someone that has been the main finance person in regards to bills in the household who now can't balance a checkbook.

There are some differences between forgetfulness and memory loss. The memory loss associated with Alzheimer's progresses more rapidly and is more readily noticeable to family and friends than forgetfulness brought on by the aging process. Age related memory loss may affect the person's ability to remember new information but typically it will not interfere with the ability to live independently and function in everyday life. Alzheimer's disease affects several areas of the brain that include the ability to reason, judgment, as well as the language abilities. Alzheimer's affects not only memory but also the ability to find the words to describe objects as well as to locate familiar places. A person with age related memory loss may have trouble remembering something, eventually will recall it, while a person with Alzheimer's rarely has this ability. Someone with Alzheimer's disease will forget complete experiences rather than parts of them.

Let's take a little time now to break down some of the words used in the above paragraphs.

What is Memory?

     Memory is the ability to store and retrieve information.

There are 3 memory systems:

    Sensory

    Short-term

    Long-term

Sensory memory receives information through the five senses and passes that information on to the short-term memory. Short term memory receives information from the sensory memory and information can stay in this memory for a short period of time, typically 15-20 seconds. Long-term memory recalls information gathered over time and the information can stay for a few days or for a lifetime. This memory processes information.

The things most likely forgotten are names, where you put something, telephone numbers, words, or having already told something to someone. Ways to compensate for memory changes include exercising regularly, have your eyes and ears checked, do memory exercises and review your medication with you doctor routinely. Possible causes of memory loss include drug intoxication, depression, head injury, dementia, or stroke.

Forgetfulness: Aging or Alzheimer's?

Activity	Age Related	Alzheimer's
Forgets	Parts of an experience	Whole experience
Remembers later	Often	Rarely
Follow written/spoken directions	Usually able	Gradually unable
Can use notes	Usually able	Gradually unable
Care for self	Usually able	Gradually unable

This gives you a little insight regarding age related memory loss and loss of memory due to the Alzheimer's process.

Dementia is the decline in mental function and is more severe than age-related difficulties. It interferes with daily activities and social relationships. It is not simply poor memory or forgetfulness.

There are many different types of dementia which we will discuss. Before we discuss the different types of dementia keep in mind that I am not giving you the complete list. I am listing a few to give you a knowledge base.

Reversible dementia is caused by a number of diseases and conditions and if treated the decline seen intellectually is reversed. About 10 to 15 percent of dementias are reversible. The causes of reversible dementia include vitamin deficiency, depression, malnutrition, infections, anemia, drugs, alcohol, hypothyroidism, brain tumors, head trauma, and medications.

Irreversible dementia results in the deterioration of intellectual functioning and is progressive and fatal. Alzheimer's disease is the most common. All of the dementias we are about to discuss are irreversible. Think of dementia and all the different types in this way: Dementia is the base of the tree and all the different types of dementia are the limbs attached to the tree.

Familial Alzheimer's is an early on-set type of Alzheimer's dementia. Diagnosis can be seen in the 30's-50's. Progress is more rapid and prognosis is only 3-7 years. Only about 5% of the dementias fall into this category. If your parents have this diagnosis you have a 50% risk as one of the children to develop the same diagnosis.

Here is a chart of a few of the irreversible types of dementia's.

Alzheimer's disease	The most common form of dementia. Fourth leading cause of death in adults, after heart disease, cancer, and stroke. It attacks the brain and affects men and women the same. More women develop disease. It results in impaired memory, thinking, and behavior and can last 3-20 years. A definite diagnosis can only be obtained through autopsy.
Multi-infarct dementia	Known as vascular dementia. It is a deterioration of mental capacity caused by multiple strokes in the brain. This may also be described as mini strokes. These strokes may damage areas of the brain responsible for a specific function as well as produce general symptoms of dementia.
Parkinson's disease	A progressive disorder of the central nervous system that affects over one million Americans. This disorder causes certain brain cells to deteriorate for unknown reasons. It is characterized by tremors, stiffness in limbs and joints, speech difficulties and difficulty with physical movement.

Huntington's disease	An inherited degenerative brain disease. It affects the mind and body. It usually begins during mid-life and is characterized by intellectual decline, irregular and involuntary movements of the limbs or facial muscles. You may also see personality change, memory disturbance, slurred speech, impaired judgment and psychiatric problems. Children born to a person with this disease have a 50% chance of inheriting the gene that causes it. There in no treatment available to stop progression but the psychiatric symptoms and movement disorders can be controlled by medications.
Creutzfeld-Jakob disease	Also known as the mad cow disease. It is a rare fatal brain disorder that causes rapid, progressive dementia and other neuromuscular disturbances. Symptoms are similiar to Alzheimer's. The only way for a definite diagnosis is through an autopsy.
Lewy Body dementia	An irreversible form of dementia associated with abnormal protein deposits in the brain called Lewy bodies. Symptoms are similar to Alzheimer's symptoms. Hallucinations and paranoia also may become more apparent than in Alzheimer's.

Now that you have learned a little about different types of irreversible dementias it is time to discuss the different stages of dementia. Dementias are classified into 3 stages which include early, middle and late stages. During the early stage you may still live at home or in an assisted living. In the middle stage more supervision is needed. Typically supervision comes from resources like home health care, non-medical care, nursing homes or assisted livings. During the last stage the individual may become bedridden and may possibly need hospice type care.

Below is a chart about the 3 stages of Alzheimer's dementia. This is only to give you an overview of what to expect. The one thing I have learned from my Alzheimer's residents is to expect the unexpected! There will not be a day when you wake up and say "mom has now entered the middle stage and she appears to be about half way through it!" Granted by educating yourself and observing them over time you can feel fairly confident on saying "Looking back on things I remember a time over 5 years ago when they started exhibiting the signs of Alzheimer's." "I did not recognize the signs at the time." The main point is to have a little idea of where they are currently and be ready to face each day with your best foot forward. Please do not get so lost in what stage they may be in that you lose one of those precious moments where they are more oriented.

Three Stages Of Alzheimer's

Early (Mild)	Middle (Moderate)	Late (Severe)
Lasts 2-4 years	Become more confused about recent events	May be unable to use or understand words
Get lost easily even in places they know well	Experience difficulty with simple daily activities	May not recognize self in a mirror
Lose interest in things they enjoyed	Last 2-10 years	Last 1-3 years
Have trouble finding names for common items	Argue more often than usual	May not recognize family members
Lose things more often than normal	Believe things are real when they are not	Can not care for themselves at all
Undergo personality changes	Often require close supervision	Lose interest in food, chewing, and swallowing difficulties
Difficulty learning new things	Display anxiety or depression	Incontinence occurs

There are many symptoms of Alzheimer's. Some of the symptoms include memory loss that affects your everyday life, poor or decreased judgment, problems naming a common object such as a pen or watch, getting lost easily even in familiar places, lack of initiative in usual activities and problems with abstract thinking. Other symptoms include changes in mood or personality, problems performing a familiar task such as using an appliance, losing or misplacing items frequently, unsure of time and place, and problems with language abilities.

Steps to diagnose someone with Alzheimer's is a process of elimination which include:

- Symptoms of dementia are present
- A medical history has been done
- Physical, neurological and psychological exam
- Appropriate lab work
- Specific diagnostic testing.

An autopsy is the only way to verify if the person has Alzheimer's. Please keep in mind that doctors still may diagnose them with Alzheimer's. If they have followed all the steps to diagnose and have ruled out any other diagnosis they may feel confident that Alzheimer's is the appropriate diagnosis.

Treatment includes non-*prescription as well as prescription*. Vitamin E, Ginkgo Biloba, and non steroidal anti-inflammatory drugs are some of the over the counter drugs available to you. Prescriptions medications include Donepezil HCl (Aricept),Tacrine HCl (Cognex),Exelon,Reminyl, and Namenda. Talk with your doctor about possibilities available in medications, side effects, and what track record the drug has on the ability to slow down Alzheimer's.

A thought to live by is what's good for the heart is good for the brain. Exercise, mental stimulation, social activity, emotional health and eating in a well balanced way.

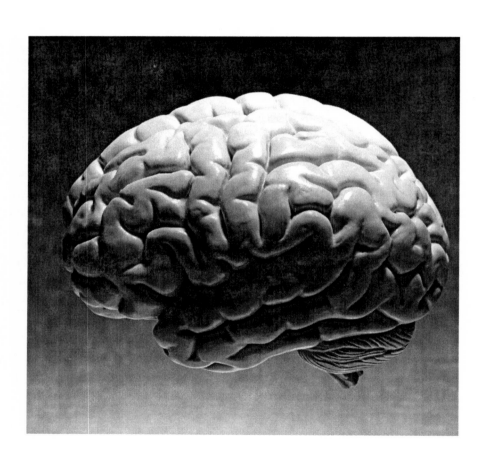

CHAPTER 7

INSIDE THE HUMAN BRAIN

Inside the human brain

The reason for learning a little bit about the brain and its function is to help you understand some of the physical differences that you may witness due to the Alzheimer's disease process. By learning about the brain you will also know that the person you are taking care of is not exhibiting certain behaviors to get your attention. Alzheimer's attacks the brain and slowly eats away at it. An inflicted brain may lose weight due to the disease attacking it and it looks like a shriveled dried up peach instead of that once juicy plumb peach.

Let's look at the three main parts of the brain which include the cerebral hemispheres, cerebellum and brain stem. The cerebral hemispheres are where sensory information is received from the outside world and is then processed. This part of the brain also controls voluntary movement and regulates conscious thought and mental activity. The cerebellum is in charge of balance and coordination and receives information from the eyes, ears, muscles and joints about body's movements and positions. Lastly, the brain stem connects the spinal cord with the brain and it relays and receives messages to and from muscles, skin and other organs. It also controls automatic functions such as heart rate, blood pressure and breathing.

There are also other important players inside the brain that include the hippocampus. This is where short-term memories are converted to long-term memories. The thalamus receives sensory and limbic information and sends to the cerebral cortex. The hypothalamus monitors certain activities and controls body's internal clock. The limbic system controls emotions and instinctive behavior.

Plaques and tangles are considered at this time the leading signs of Alzheimer's. The brains of people with Alzheimer's have an abundance of two abnormal structures which include the beta-amyloid plaques and the neurofiblrillary tangles. Beta-amyloid plaques are dense deposits of protein and cellular material that accumulate outside and around nerve cells. Beta-amyloid fragments come together in clumps to form plaques. Neurofibrillary tangles are twisted fibers that build up inside the nerve cell. In Alzheimer's many of these clumps form, disrupting the work of neurons. This affects the hippocampus and other areas of the cerebral cortex.

No one knows what causes Alzheimer's, but we do know a lot about what happens in the brain once it starts to unfold in the brain. Signs of Alzheimer's are first noticed in the entorhinal cortex and then proceed to the hippocampus. The affected regions begin to shrink as nerve cells die. Changes can begin 10-20 years before symptoms appear. Memory loss is the first sign of Alzheimer's. Alzheimer's disease spreads through the brain. The cerebral cortex begins to shrink as more and more neurons stop working and die. Death usually occurs from aspiration pneumonia or other infections.

Through all of this clinical education that you are receiving there is one important concept to walk away with. This disease is attacking the brain and the abilities of the person you are taking care of are going to deteriorate over time. It will not only affect their memory but also their communication abilities, behaviors, physical abilities and personality. This disease will progressively worsen with time and is like a spiraling down staircase.

Normal(left)   Alzheimer's (right)

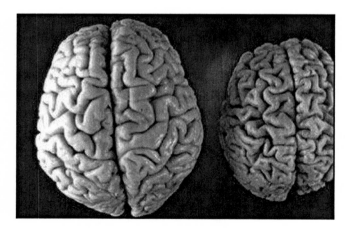

NOTES

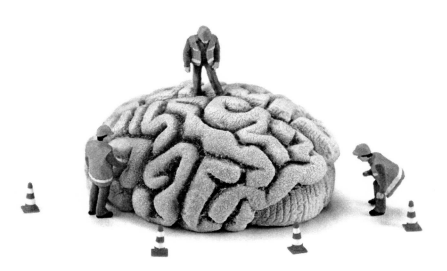

64

CHAPTER 8

RESEARCH

Research

Research on many aspects of Alzheimer's disease is underway around the world. In the United States the National Institute on Aging (NIA), part of the National Institutes of Health, leads the way in federal funding for research on Alzheimer's disease. Other organizations, including the Alzheimer's Association, also fund many types of Alzheimer's research.

Most organizations that provide money to researchers also make research findings available to anyone who is interested. You can find articles and news about the latest research findings through these organizations and through groups that focus on education and advocacy. Information on how to contact these organizations to learn more or to participate in research studies is found in the resource chapter.

Finding a cure for Alzheimer's disease will require a better understanding of the cause or causes of the disease. Researchers who study causes and cures use a number of strategies. One common strategy is to create situations in cells or in animals that are similar to those of a human with Alzheimer's disease. These are called "models" of Alzheimer's disease. Ideas about causes and cures can be tested in these models. Sometimes the models allow researchers to ask questions that cannot be answered with research on humans.

Although scientists are still searching for clues as to what causes Alzheimer's disease, they do know some of the risk factors for the disease. It is important to remember that risk factors are not the same as causes. For example, older age is a well-known risk factor for late-onset Alzheimer's disease. This means that persons are more likely to get the disease as they get older, but it does not mean that age causes the disease.

Genetics play a role in Alzheimer's disease, although the exact role is not fully understood. Genes like apolipoprotein E-e4 (APOE-e4) seem to be associated with the disease. The AD Genetics Study, funded by NIA, is one example of the many studies that are currently underway to learn more about the roles of genetics and family history in Alzheimer disease (www.ncrad.org).

Scientists are looking to see if Alzheimer's disease can be prevented or delayed by changing some of the risk factors that we can control. These factors include physical health, social relationships, stress, and cognitive activity like challenging ourselves to learn new things. The National Institutes of Health and the Centers for Disease Control are funding efforts to promote brain health among older adults. Scientists are also studying different approaches to prevention, which include drugs that protect cells in the brain from damage that may lead to the disease.

In recent years there have been some important advances in technologies that may help with the development of medications to treat Alzheimer's disease and with earlier diagnosis. Examples of these technologies include special compounds that bind to plaques and tangles in the brain. These plaques and tangles are changes in the cells of the brain that are associated with Alzheimer's disease. When compounds bind to the plaques and tangles, it is easier to see these brain changes using neuroimaging techniques like PET or MRI scans. Compounds like FDDNP and Pittsburgh Compound B are helpful in determining whether medications reduce the plaques and tangles associated with Alzheimer's disease. Eventually, they may help physicians diagnose Alzheimer's disease earlier.

Researchers are continuing to look for drugs that can ease the symptoms and slow the progress of Alzheimer's disease. There is much interest in finding drugs and other interventions that can be used for persons with Mild Cognitive Impairment (MCI). Persons with MCI have cognitive impairments that usually appear as mild memory problems. MCI is not the same as Alzheimer's disease, but it is a risk factor for Alzheimer's disease. We can learn about the causes and possible treatments of the disease by studying MCI. It may be possible to prevent some cases of Alzheimer's disease by treating MCI. Research into these possibilities is underway.

Scientists are looking for tools that improve the health and well-being of persons who have Alzheimer's disease. One approach has been the development of therapeutic activities like communication tools, memory training techniques, and enjoyable recreation. Research has shown that persons with Alzheimer's disease benefit from meaningful activities when those activities are customized to fit their interests and strengths. Activity-based tools are available to persons with Alzheimer's disease, families and care centers through a number of sources with some located in Chapter 9 of this book.

Caregiving for persons with dementia is a popular area of research. This includes caregiving by family members at home and professional caregiving in healthcare and residential settings. Negative effects of stress related to caring for a family member with dementia have been identified. Positive effects of caregiving have also been identified. There is evidence that skills training, stress management techniques, and social support can ease some of the negative effects of caregiving, which are likely due to both the worry and the physical work associated with providing care. Research findings also provide evidence that persons from different racial or ethnic groups seem to have different caregiving experiences.

There is evidence from research studies that staff development interventions can improve the quality of care provided by professional caregivers. In general, these interventions provide professional caregivers like nursing assistants, LVNs/LPNs and nurses with skills for communicating with persons who have Alzheimer's disease and for managing challenging behaviors of persons with Alzheimer's disease. These behaviors, which are a common symptom of Alzheimer's disease and other dementias, are thought to be due to needs that the person with dementia cannot clearly communicate and cannot meet on his or her own. Meeting these needs is one focus of staff development interventions for professional caregivers who work with persons who have Alzheimer's disease.

The examples of research related to Alzheimer's disease in this chapter are only a few highlights of the important research being conducted around the world. New findings are available every day. Organizations that fund research, educate the public and advocate for persons affected by Alzheimer's disease are a good source of information about what we know about Alzheimer's disease. They are also a good source of information on how to get involved by volunteering to participate in research studies. You can find some of these organizations listed in Chapter 9.

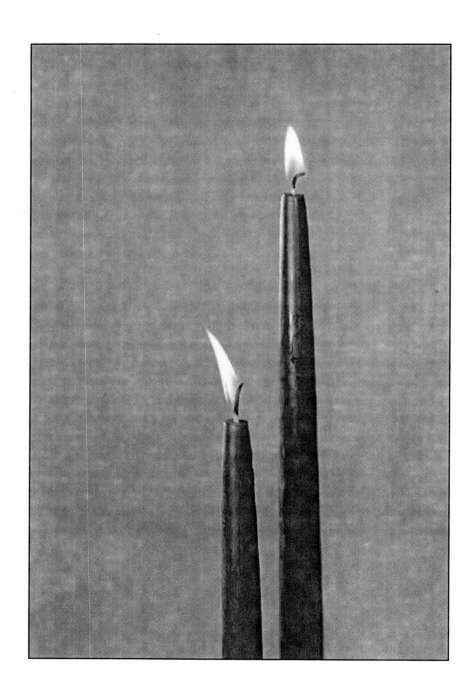

CHAPTER 9

RESOURCES

Resources

There are so many resources available to you and your loved one facing Alzheimer's. Look into support groups in your area and find the one that you feel most comfortable with. Also research daily care for Alzheimer's referred to as adult day care. Another resource to check into is the safe return program offered through the Alzheimer's Association. The safe return program offers you peace of mind by offering a bracelet with information to help find your loved one if they become displaced from you.

Where Can I Find More Information about Research and Alzheimer's Disease and other resources?

Organization/Source	Contact Information
National Institute on Aging (NIA)	www.nia.nih.gov
Alzheimer's Association	www.alz.org/800-272-3900
Alzheimer's Disease Education & Referral Center	www.nia.nih.gov/alzheimers 800-438-4380
Alzheimer's Foundation of America	www.alzfdn.org
Alzheimer's Disease Cooperative Study	Adcs.ucsd.edu
National Library of Medicine's PubMed search service	www.ncbi.nlm.nih.gov/entrez/
AD Genetics Study	www.ncrad.org 1-800-526-2839
Cognitive and Emotional Health Project	Trans.nih.gov/CEHP/
CDC Healthy Brain Initiative	www.cdc.gov/aging/healthybrain.htm#1
Alzheimer's Disease Neuroimaging Initiative	www.loni.ucla.edu/ADNI/
Myers Research Institute	www.myersresearch.org
Family Caregiver Alliance	www.caregiver.org

Rosalyn Carter Institute for Caregiving	www.rosalyncarter.org
REACH (Resources for Enhancing Alzheimer's Caregiver Health)	www.edc.gsph.pitt.edu/reach/
National Clearinghouse on the Direct Care Workforce	www.directcareclearinghouse.org

MEDICAID HOTLINE   1-800-252-8263

Toll-free number for general information and counseling on Medicaid.

http://cms.hhs.gov/
Web site for Medicaid and Medicare Services (formerly called Health Care Financing Administration).
General information on Medicaid and Medicare.

MEDICARE   1-800-633-4227

National toll-free number for general information and counseling on

Medicare.

www.medicare.gov
Official U.S. government site for Medicare information on eligibility, enrollment, and premiums.
Search tools for state-specific information on health plan choices; nursing home comparisons; prescription drug programs; participating physicians; and plan coverage.

OFFICE OF THE ATTORNEY GENERAL   1-800-621-0508
CONSUMER PROTECTION DIVISION
Register complaints against businesses; report senior fraud.
www.oag.state.tx.us/elder/elder.shtml
Senior Texans' page includes information on consumer protection; rights of the elderly; choosing a nursing home; advance planning; health and safety; and Senior Alerts.

www.Reminisce Magazine.com

Creative Forecasting at www.creativeforecasting.net

Mind and Memory Store at www.mindandmemory.com

Nasco: Senior Activities 800-558-9595/www.eNasco.com/
senoiractivities

AARP(American Association of Retried Persons) 888-687-2277/
www.aarp.org

Family Caregiver Alliance 800-445-8106/www.caregiver.org

Children of Aging Parents 800-227-7294/www.caps4caregivers.org

Texas Department of Protective and Regulatory Services 1-800-252-
5400 Hotline for reporting abuse, neglect, or exploitation of children,
the elderly or people with disabilities. Available 24/7.

Elder Options of Texas/ www.elderoptionsoftexas.com

Legal Hotline for Older Texans 1-800-622-2520 Legal assistance
including counseling, representation, and document preparation.

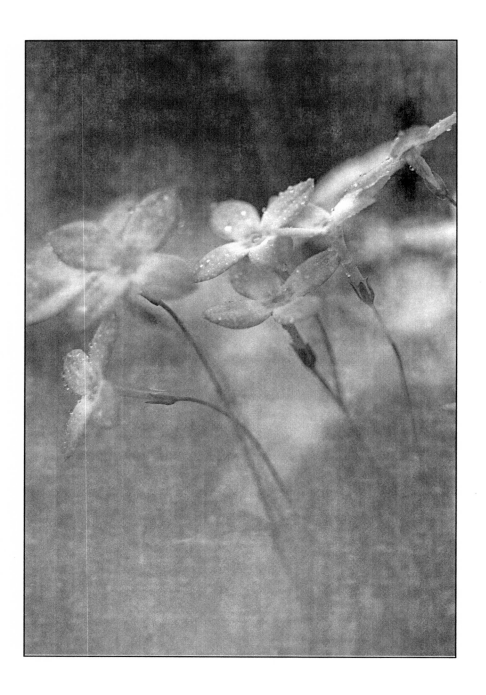

Chapter 10

Forget Me Knots

FORGET ME KNOTS

This chapter titled Forget Me Knots is exactly that. I will discuss aspects of Alzheimer's and health related items that you as the caregiver may overlook while trying to keep the day to day activities going. I will discuss Prearrangement, in home care, Assisted Livings (general as well as Alzheimer's specific), sexuality and other aspects that you need to keep in mind during your caregiving life with Alzheimer's.

The first one to discuss is **Prearrangement**. I chose to discuss this one first because it is very important and we as a society do not like to talk about death. I am going to ask you to shop for your loved one's death as well as your own death. In the event of your death, would your family know what to do? The death of a loved one is one of the most traumatic and trying times in anyone's life. You and your family can be overwhelmed by the sense of loss, grief and confusion not to mention the legal and financial details. Funeral decisions involving important questions of appropriateness, desirability and affordability are even more difficult at the time of death. All too often, this is exactly when these important, difficult questions must be made, and by those who are already under a great deal of stress. Although we know that death is inevitable we don't like to think about it. We especially don't like to plan for it. Thus the burden is thrust upon family members to make decisions that may be inappropriate or wasteful and may not reflect our own personal desires.

By making your funeral arrangements now, you can spare your loved ones the burden of having to do it under stressful conditions. Pre-arranging can help make a difficult time a little easier on those you care so much about and you are insured that your own personal wishes are made known.

When you plan your funeral arrangements in advance you're giving your family more than just a record of your service wishes. You're also telling them how much they mean to you. Planning ahead takes so little time, yet it gives your family what they'll need most: Time together and time to heal. You are giving your loved ones their last gift!

Reasons and advantages of pre-arrangements include the decision process and fiscal burden are lightened. This is a part of thorough estate planning. It allows the opportunity to answer questions relating to types of services, costs and alternatives that are available. Decisions are not hastily made and are reached without anxiety. Usually there are no obligations or costs involved for a consultation with a Pre-arrangement counselor. This consultation can take place in the intimacy of your home or in the comfort of the funeral home of your choice. Give your family one last gift at your death by choosing to prearrange!

Non-medical homecare(personal sitter group) is care that takes place in the home of a senior that fulfills a variety of needs ranging from assistance with activities of daily living such as bathing, dressing, grooming, and toileting assistance to more basic household duties such as light housekeeping, meal preparation and transportation. Care plans are typically devised on a weekly schedule and are tailored to best meet the needs of the individual care recipient.

There are several things to look for when selecting a homecare agency that will provide the best possible care for a loved one. Ask if criminal backgrounds checks are performed on all employees of the personal sitter group of your choice. Additionally, the opportunity to meet with caregivers prior to actual care beginning is an important guarantee of superior caregivers. You can also find some personal caregiving agencies that specialize in Alzheimer's care by offering extra education to their staff as well as a structured activity schedule to help assist loved ones in their journey.

Finally, several other factors should be looked at when selecting a homecare agency and determining if non-medical homecare is right for a loved one. Any agency that is used should be licensed by the State of Texas Department of Human Services. Also, an agency in question should possess general liability as well as bonding insurance. Finally, learning about the on call policy of an agency can be extremely important to determine how available backup caregivers are going to be if sickness or other issues prevent the regular caregiver from performing care during the established care plan. Always reevaluate your agency of choice periodically to make sure it is a good fit for you and your loved one.

Home health and hospice are also available in the home setting. These options may work in your home setting along with a personal sitter group or as a stand alone. Watch your loved one for exit seeking and wandering types of behaviors and stay realistic in regards to how many hours your support systems are helping you throughout each day.

Another option is home health and hospice offering their services within an assisted living.

Finding an **Assisted Living** right for you can prove to be a difficult task due to the complex nature of the services Assisted Living communities provide and the large variation in facilities that offer these services. In general, an Assisted Living facility furnishes food and shelter to four or more persons who are unrelated to the owner of the establishment and provides personal care services. Assisted Living services are driven by a service philosophy that emphasizes personal dignity, autonomy, independence and privacy. They should enhance a person's ability to age in place in a residential setting while receiving increasing or decreasing levels of service as the person's needs change.

Any resident that resides in a Type A licensed facility must be physically and mentally capable of evacuating the facility unassisted, does not require routine attendance during nighttime sleeping hours, and must be capable of following directions under emergency conditions.

A resident residing in a Type B licensed facility may require staff assistance to evacuate, may be incapable of following directions under emergency conditions, may require attendance during nighttime sleeping hours, or may not be permanently bedfast, but may require assistance in transferring to and from a wheelchair.

A great starting point to obtain information about a facility is in their display case. Assisted Living facilities are required to post their current license, which will tell you if they are licensed as Type A or B, small or large. They must post the most current state inspection which will list all, if any, deficiencies found in the total operation of the facility. The Assisted Living Disclosure Statement contains information regarding the preadmission, admission and discharge process, resident assessment and service plans, staffing patterns, the physical environment of the facility, resident activities, and facility services. You may ask for a copy of the Disclosure Statement if you wish.

When looking for an Assisted Living for your loved one with Alzheimer's there are some extra things that you need to think about before making your final decision. First, look for an Assisted Living that is completely secured for your loved ones protection. Research this in more detail. Some doors will open after you push on them for 15 seconds while others are truly completely secure. Another important aspect to notice is if your loved one will have access to outside at all times in a secure way. Everyone enjoys and needs to be outside at times. Agitation can also increase if there is not access to the outside available at all times. Look for an Assisted Living that specializes in Alzheimer's if available in your area. Typically, an Assisted Living specializing in Alzheimer's will offer more staff training, more education for the caregivers, activities that are Alzheimer's appropriate as well as a failure free environment. Whether you decide on a general Assisted Living or a specialized Alzheimer's home remember that bigger is not always better. Bigger areas including living, bedroom and closet space can overwhelm and set your loved one up for failure which can lead to more behaviors. Look for professionals that you are comfortable with and feel that you can talk with. There is no Assisted Living that you are truly going to be happy with because you will not be the one offering the care to your own loved one. The Assisted Living will at times make mistakes so it is important to have an open line of communication so you can work through things together. If Assisted Living ends up not being a good fit and you need to look at nursing homes the same general guidelines apply.

Financial and legal planning is another area that society as a whole does not like to discuss with others. Listed are a few key points that you need to handle no matter what. The first item to take care of is a Will. Almost 70% of adults do not have a Will in place. A Will can be quick and easy to do. You need to name an executor and you need to be as detailed as possible in regards to your property. You can research drawing up a Will online or find a lawyer to help you. You also need a Durable Power of Attorney (POA) to cover medical as well as financial. Without a POA families can be faced with becoming their loved ones guardian which is not only financially draining but also will cause emotional turmoil. If you become the guardian your loved one loses their legal rights as a person and this can be emotionally difficult to swallow.

A Do Not Resuscitate (DNR) order is a type of advanced directive. A DNR is an order to not have CPR administered if your heart stops beating or if you stop breathing. Another type of advanced directive is a Living Will. This type comes into to play when you are terminally ill and generally means you have less than 6 months to live. You can describe the kind of treatment you would like. It does not allow you to appoint someone to make medical decisions for you. It is the medical POA that does that.

Sexuality is another topic that is forgotten about when the diagnosis of Alzheimer's has been given. The spouse caregiver along with their loved one diagnosed with Alzheimer's are faced with yet another obstacle. We all have a need for companionship and physical intimacy. People with Alzheimer's disease are no different in regards to this human need.

The changes in the brain brought about by the disease process can increase their need for sexual relations which can create an uncomfortable situation for all involved. Others with the disease may have less of a sex drive and interest due to depression. There are medications to help with both extremes of sexuality. It is important to remember that changes in sexual behavior are not a reflection of character but are symptoms of the disease.

The changes in the relationship can be frustrating for both partners. The partner with Alzheimer's may show less inhibitions then before and may say or do things that their partner feels is inappropriate. The brain controls our inhibitions and if the disease has eaten that area away you may see more inappropriate sexual behaviors. If you are dealing with an inappropriate sexual behavior avoid becoming angry, do not express shock and do not ridicule your loved one. Try gentle reminders that the behavior is not appropriate.

Partners may feel guilty and may not know how to respond to their loved one anymore. You may also not find your loved one sexually appealing due to your new caregiving role. It is important to try to meet your needs for companionship and physical intimacy with your partner with Alzheimer's in a way that encourages respect and dignity for both partners.

As the disease progresses, your loved one with Alzheimer's may not recognize you. You will need a great deal of support and understanding from others. The caregiver is also faced with the concern that their loved one with Alzheimer's may find a "new" partner due to not remembering you even if you have been their husband for the last 60 years. This is seen more in a long term care setting. These types of relationships that occur in long term care settings are not typically of the sexual nature. More often you will see hand holding or a kiss on the cheek. This is still difficult for the caregiver partner to understand so it is important to ensure that an agreement and understanding of the new relationship is made no matter what form it takes.

While dealing with the issues that inappropriate sexual behavior may bring along with the concern or realization that your loved one does not recognize you any longer keep one main stay in mind. Take care of yourself. Only you can determine what that will mean for you. You are in a very delicate situation and during your struggles within reach out to the support systems around you for guidance and advice.

Driving is another huge obstacle that you face with your loved one with Alzheimer's. It is very difficult for many loved ones to take the keys away from their loved one. Overall, someone with Alzheimer's and driving a vehicle is not a good combination. The disease affects memory loss, disorientation, shortened attention span, impaired judgment and spatial perception impairment. Driving will become very dangerous for themselves, their passengers and others on the road.

Evaluate your loved ones ability to drive regularly. If any of the following problems are experienced you may need to limit or stop their driving completely.

1. Do they get lost while traveling to a familiar location?
2. Do they make slow or poor decisions?
3. Do they drive at inappropriate speeds? Too fast or slow?
4. Do they observe traffic signals?
5. Do they become confused, frustrated or angry while driving?

If any of these above signs are noticed please take immediate action. Do not wait for an accident to occur!

Talking with them about no longer being able to drive can be very difficult. The loss of the ability to drive represents a loss of independence to anyone. They may exhibit denial, grief or anger over your decision. You will need to remain consistent and firm with your decision. If you are having troubles implementing this by yourself involve their primary doctor. Doctors are a great support in regards to this obstacle. Many states have laws requiring physicians to report Alzheimer's dementia and related disorders to the Department of Motor Vehicles. The Department of Motor Vehicles then has the responsibility of retesting the driver with Alzheimer's. There are approaches to use if they are adamant that they are going to drive. For example: Tell them the doctor has prescribed that they no longer can drive and have the doctor write a prescription that states "Do not drive." Ask the doctor to write the Department of Motor Vehicles about situation and their inability to continue driving and keep a copy of the letter to show them. Try to walk when possible or offer to drive. Move the vehicle off of their property to your own home or a friend's house. Try hiding the car keys or give them a set of keys that do not go with their vehicle. You may want to consider selling the vehicle and put the money from the sale towards repairs, insurance, medical bills, etc. Never leave them alone in a parked car due to the fact that they may decide to get behind the wheel and drive off!

Taking the car keys away from your loved one is one of the first steps you will encounter in your changing role as a caregiver. You will continue to see yourself more in a parental role along with your everyday caregiver roles. The "parental" role is very difficult for many caregivers to embrace. Remember to take it day by day and failure can not occur as long as you never give up!

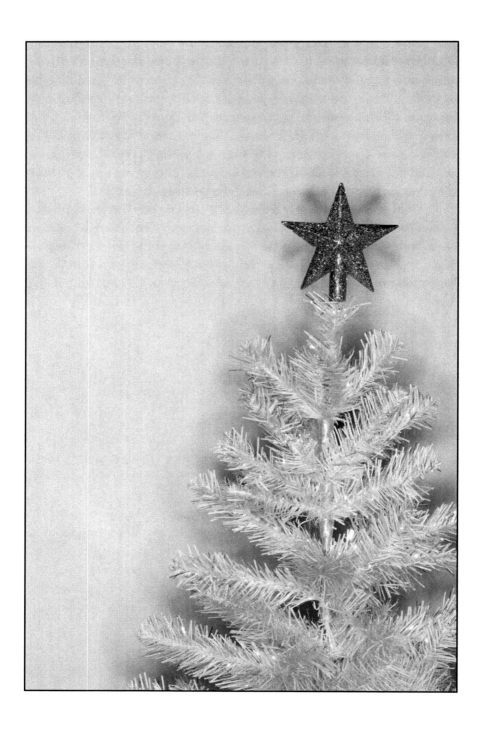

Chapter 11

Hope For Holidays

Hope For Holidays

Holidays are a tough and stressful time on the caregiver as well as the person with Alzheimer's. As a caregiver you may feel overwhelmed with all the holiday traditions you are trying to maintain on top of taking care of the person with Alzheimer's. It is also difficult to make decisions about sharing the holiday time with friends and family due to the behavioral changes that may have occurred in your loved one. As the caregiver you may feel more guilt, frustration and anger during the holiday season. All these feelings are normal and other caregivers experience the same.

You can make the holiday season a good experience for everyone involved by adjusting what you typically expect from the holiday season. Follow a few simple steps and your stress will be alleviated.

1. Discuss holiday celebrations with relatives and close friends to ensure that there is an understanding of the loved one's current situation and that expectations are realistic.
2. Only do what you can. Have a potluck type meal and invite fewer people.
3. Send out a letter to your loved ones prior to the visit to let them know how things are going currently. Go into detail on your loved one's memory and include some tips on how to communicate, any behavioral issues that they may notice, and ask them to call before arrival.

Preparation for the holiday can include your loved one. Give safe and manageable activities. Some examples include wrapping gifts, preparation of the food, decorating tree with you, singing holiday songs, setting the table or any other traditions or ideas you may have. Maintain a normal routine and keep the tasks at a level that will not overwhelm or confuse your loved one. Tree with blinking lights, loud singing/music, loud crowds and loud TV can cause confusion and behavior in your loved one. Avoid flashy lights and loud noises if at all possible. Also avoid candles, poinsettias and artificial fruit. Encourage useful gift buying for your loved one, examples include photo albums, videos of loved ones, favorite music and favorite movies. If you are receiving gifts ask for gift certificates to places that would pamper you. For example: your favorite restaurant, massage, pedicure, etc.

If your loved one is in a nursing home or assisted living do a trial run before the holiday season and see how well it goes. If home visits are too stressful try visits in small groups at your loved one's nursing home or assisted living.

Traveling can be another obstacle to overcome. If you need to travel make sure you have your loved one has some sort of ID showing that they have Alzheimer's. The Alzheimer's Association has a program called the Safe Return Program-ID bracelet. Put ID cards with photo and phone numbers in several of your loved one's pockets. Never leave your loved one alone not even for a second! Have a plan for toileting if a different gender. Try to find family or friends to travel with to increase the safety factor. Have a plan in place for emergency purposes. If staying in a hotel/motel secure the room door completely, purchase an inexpensive door alarm and try to keep the daily routine comparable. If your car is not equipped with child proof door locks rent a newer car that has this feature. Make sure you leave a detailed itinerary with family and friends. Check in and let them know if you will be changing your plans in anyway.

You will have post-holiday let down so prepare for this also. Have plans after the holidays to enjoy yourself in some way to alleviate the stress and let down that you are feeling. Take many breaks and try to keep your daily routine the same as much as possible.

NOTES

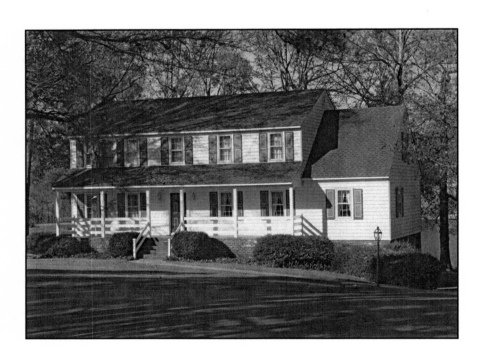

Chapter 12

Home Safety

HOME SAFETY

Home safety is crucial in regards to Alzheimer's. Many of us continue to choose to keep our loved one in the home for as long as possible. In this chapter home safety with dignity and security will be discussed. Plus you will be able to sleep better at night and have peace of mind.

In general while safe proofing your home always keep 3 key points in mind:

1. Change the environment if needed
2. Think of prevention and be proactive
3. Danger, Danger, Danger

Leaving your loved one alone can be a difficult decision to make. Some things to ask yourself when making this decision include but are not limited to the following:

1. Do they show signs of confusion during stressful situations?
2. Do they know how to get help if needed?
3. Do they know if they are is in danger? For example: A fire in the home.
4. Do they know how to use a phone during an emergency?
5. Do they still try to cook, smoke, or other hobbies that may need an appliance that is plugged in?
6. Do they have wandering or exit seeking moments?
7. Do they become depressed or angry when left alone?

You may want to discuss with other family members as well as their primary doctor to help you make the decision in regards to being alone.

You will need to go room by room and do a safety check of each room looking for potential hazards.Take proactive measures to ensure your loved one's safety. During your room to room check here are 50 concerns and/or suggestions to keep in mind.

1. Do you have smoke detectors and carbon monoxide detectors in appropriate areas of the home? Don't forget to do maintenance checks periodically along with a battery check.
2. The phone ringing can be overwhelming and frustrating for your loved one so have your answering machine pick up with

fewest rings possible. Also answering the phone may put your loved one in a failure type environment due to not being able to take a message.

3. Have emergency numbers as well as your home address posted near each phone for emergency use for yourself as well as your loved one.

4. Secure all doors and windows so they can not put themselves in an unsafe situation during a disoriented moment.

5. Keep all your pathways clear for tripping hazards. Examples of tripping hazards include loose rugs and extension cords. If you must use extension cords keep them close to your baseboards.

6. Keep a spare key hidden just in case you get locked out of the home.

7. Cover unused outlets with childproof plugs.

8. Stairways should have handrails with carpet or safety grips on the stairs.

9. Fish tanks are not a good idea due to glass, water, potential poisonous life and electrical pumps. This is not a good combination.

10. Power tools and other machinery in the garage or storage buildings should be locked up.

11. Remove all poisonous type landscape or flowers from your home.

12. Keep alcohol locked up.

13. Keep medications locked up.

14. Keep cleaning supplies locked up or out of reach.

15. Remove all guns and ammunition or keep locked up and out of reach.

16. If they smoke all smoking materials should be locked up and taken out for them to smoke. Never allow them to smoke alone.

17. If you have a computer in the home and have things you do not want deleted password protect them or save them on a thumb type drive and lock up the thumb drive.

18. Avoid clutter and keep plastic bags out of reach due to suffocation and choking hazard.

19. Remove the fuel source to grills as well as the lighting devices.

20. Lock up swimming area if applicable.

21. Install childproof door latches on storage cabinets and drawers.
22. You may want a NO SOLICITING sign for the front door.
23. Lock up knives and other sharp devices.
24. Keep small appliances out of reach.
25. Remove knobs from stove and possibly an automatic shut off switch.
26. Take a look at your "junk" drawer. We all have one. Secure all small type items out of their reach.
27. Remove artificial fruits, veggies or magnets in shape of fruits or veggies to ensure they do not mistake for real food and try to eat.
28. You may want to dismantle the garbage disposal.
29. Have night lights throughout your home.
30. Have intercom type devices throughout home (baby monitors) to monitor other rooms.
31. Do not use portable space heaters.
32. Do not use electric blankets or heating pads.
33. Remove locks from bathrooms and bedrooms so they can not lock themselves in on accident.
34. Have nonskid strips in the bathtub and shower area.
35. Look at having grab bars in the toilet and tub area.
36. Use shower chair if needed.
37. Adjust your water heater to 120 degrees to avoid scalding.
38. Remove remote controls in the living room.
39. Do not have a fire in the fireplace.
40. Keep all vehicles securely locked.
41. Make sure all doors to outside have locks that are not at eyelevel. Invest in door alarms to alert you if they open a door to the outside.
42. Place Stop, Do Not Enter, or Closed signs on doors to the outside.
43. Enroll in the Safe Return program through the Alzheimer's Association.
44. Place labels in clothing with identification
45. Keep a set of worn clothing in a plastic bag for police dog to help find them if this is ever needed.
46. Educate your neighbors on their potential to wander and to

become disoriented.

47. Have recent pictures of her available for neighbors, family and police if they do get lost.

48. Keep trashcan out of sight and check for items that may have been thrown away by accident.

49. Avoid violent or disturbing TV shows. DVD's of shows they enjoyed many years ago is your best bet.

50. Keep spices locked up due to harmful ingestion of too much of a spice.

Take this list a bit at a time and implement what you feel is most important for your loved ones situation. It does not need to be done all in one day. Work on it a bit each day and before you know it you will have everything done and even found other areas of concerns not listed in the above list.

NOTES

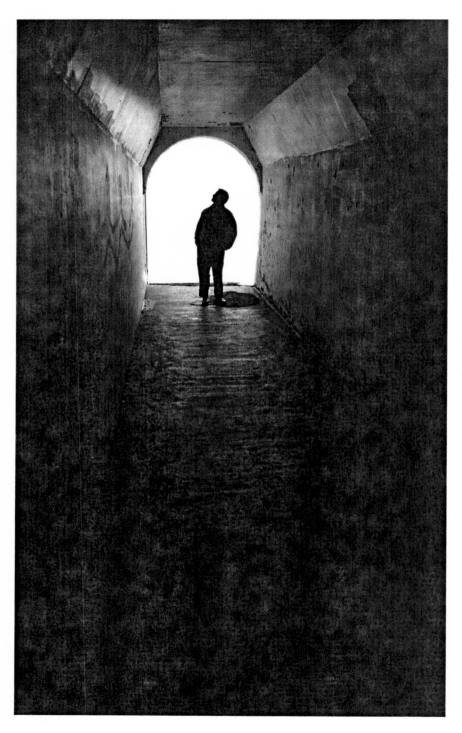

CHAPTER 13

LIGHT IN THE TUNNEL STORIES

LIGHT IN THE TUNNEL STORIES

The stories you are about to read are true. The hope I have, along with the caregivers that submitted these stories, is to help you find a light in your tunnel. I have not changed the stories in hopes that one if not all the stories will show you light in the time of your need.

Papa

Papa was a gentle kind soul. He enjoyed farming, family and getting together with friends for a good game of 42 dominoes. He was retired from construction work when I came into his family as his daughter-in-law.

We began to see changes in Papa in the late 1980's. He would forget simple things-the name of an old friend or where he put something. We simply thought it was age related memory loss.

Papa was admitted to a long-term care facility in the fall of 1992. He could no longer care for himself. Papa would forget to eat, take his medicine and even forget how to get somewhere.

I had a hard time accepting that Papa was no longer the vibrant self-sufficient man he once was. I thought as a nurse I should know what was happening, how to deal with it and how to help the rest of the family cope. I soon found myself overwhelmed with it all. As a professional working in the long-term care field, I couldn't believe that I would experience the same stages of adjustment just the same as any other family member would. I went through shock, denial and depression just like the rest of the family did. As Papa's Alzheimer's progressed to the late middle stage into the end stage, I grew to hate the name of Alzheimer's. I did finally find acceptance before the end of his life. I was with Papa when he took his last breath and I was able to say goodbye with the knowledge he no longer had to remain in a world of confusion.

I will always remember Papa's half crooked smile and his sense of humor. I was always touched by the fact that each time he saw me he would smile and say, "There's my girl!"

As I found my light in the tunnel so can you!

A Day to Early

There was a gentleman in a nursing home that received a Haldol injection every afternoon because he would become so agitated. Staff talked with family about his behavior of always saying "I was a day too early." As the day would progress he would become more and more agitated as he made this statement. Staff found out that he had been in World War I in a very scary area and was one of a few to return from that area. This is how he ended up in the war. He lived in a small community and had his wife but no children. His homestead had the water supply for the community as well as food through his farming. He had applied with Uncle Sam due to this to allow him to not go to war. He had been told that he would not have to go because so many lives relied on him. He went into town one day to sell his eggs and check his mail. In the mail was a letter from Uncle Sam requesting his loyalty to join the service. Being a good citizen he went to the recruiting center and explained that he was waiting on paperwork that would allow him to stay in the states. The recruiter informed him that he needed to sign up because he had received the letter stating this. The man signed up and then went and told his wife and community members that relied on him that he had to leave tomorrow. He returned the next day to leave and checked his mail before leaving. In the mail was the letter from Uncle Sam giving him his reprieve to not join the service. The man took this letter to the recruiter to show him and he was told it was null and void because he had voluntarily signed up! Needless to say he went to war. Staff implemented validation therapy with this gentleman. When he started his "I was a day too early" the staff would talk with him about what had happened and how upset he must have been. Keep in mind they did this every time he started this conversation. Over time he was able to be taken off the Haldol injections and did not become near as agitated. It took a bit but we found some relief for the resident , the resident's family and for the staff.

MY DADDY BILL

It probably began in 1984 or so that Daddy Bill, my father in law, began to fall asleep on the fireplace hearth while talking to the family. We all just thought he was tired. He would misplace his billfold and think that one of us must have stolen it. Honestly we thought he was kidding us. He would go to get in the car next to the one we were all sitting in waiting for him to drive us to the country club; now that IS a scary thought. In those days not everyone was aware of the signs of Alzheimer's and most families didn't discuss it nor was the patient prescribed medications for it.

Well, things only got worse. My husband was acting as his ranch foreman at the time and would come home with story after story of milk from the grocery store left on the back of the car overnight. Cereal was strewn around the kitchen as if someone had thrown the box of cereal to try to hit the bowl. Of course the milk was outside on the car so there was no milk in the kitchen. Mail and bills would all be in the garbage can, unpaid and mixed with garbage. One day the Cadillac was suspended over a cliff as Daddy Bill had backed out of the garage and caught in on rocks before descending the cliff, thank goodness.

While working at the ranch, Daddy Bill would go to open the gate for Brent, my husband, and instead of locking it back in place; he would lock the lock to the gate. Therefore the bulls could get into the cows pasture. That is one thing a rancher would never, ever do. One day Daddy Bill was caught trying to break into his own ranch house by tearing the door off. When Brent stopped him, he became very angry. The door was not locked.

One time Brent came home furious with his Dad as Daddy Bill had accused him of soaking him with a hose, however, that couldn't have been as no one was around him at the time. Thus, Brent had had it!!

Again, things only got worse. Not once but twice, Daddy Bill was picked up driving the wrong way on IH 35 in the middle of the night. He was found fishing one night in his neighborhood on a bridge, albeit, no fishing pole. We got a call during one night from the Georgetown police department saying that they had Bill in a hotel with a shotgun, 2 poodles and just in his underwear and he was drunk. Even the police didn't know he had Alzheimer's but he didn't drink.

Finally one night Bee, his wife, called Brent and his brother to come to her aid and get their dad and take him somewhere. When they got there she was locked in their guest house with bars on the windows. So we came to have Daddy Bill at our house with our family of 6.

I began a search for a nursing home for Daddy Bill. That is one experience I will never forget. A horror I wish on no other human should have to experience. Finally I found one that was wonderful... only 4 miles from our house. That was the beginning of the Light in the Tunnel. The staff was wonderful. They were the very first ones to help us to understand that Daddy Bill was suffering from Alzheimer's.

We took Daddy Bill there one day telling him he was going to a hotel and he was perfectly happy. I cannot tell you the relief we felt knowing that someone qualified would be taking care of him.

As a foot note, Bee, his wife came to live with us on our property in a little house we built for her. However, because no one ever asked her what happened between she and Bill we never knew why after over 50 years of marriage, she never went to see him. They died 90 days apart; even though they had not seen each other since the day his sons came to get him.

Remembering

I don't remember when it stopped hurting. For that matter, I do not remember when it started. All that I know is that it hurt, for what seemed to be an eternity. The loss was shared by an entire family but the pain was very personal.

My mother, like so many other mothers, was attractive, vital, happy, energetic, and always ready to face life with strength. A teenager during the Depression and a young bride at the onset of WW II, she was small and petite but mighty. For all of her 50's, 60's and early 70's, she seemed indestructible. We all marveled at her capacity to do whatever, whenever she wanted. We admired and envied her energy. "It" was first noticed around 74. We cannot know when it began. During the brief weeks or short months that passed between visits, she seemed to change, slow, dull in small but noticeable ways. Perhaps through denial or ignorance, the family decided she had a series of "little strokes" as if that was an acceptable answer for what was occurring before our very eyes. In a brief period of time, what was petite became fragile, what was small became tiny.

Other medical conditions related to lifelong smoking suddenly reared their ugly heads and bit-by-bit began to claim her. Then at long last, the final and seemingly most cruel diagnosis came to pass, Alzheimer's. She knew, we knew, and it truly became the beginning of the end. At the point of diagnosis, she shut down. The progress of Alzheimer's was well known in my family and added to other physical challenges, we decided on no plan of action other than waiting.

Unlike so many who travail with this terrible disease for years, we did not experience the average 8-12 years of personal and family heartache. The fact that it went quickly, just a couple of years, did not make it easy.

With my father and his cancer, we had time...Time to grow closer, share memories, and spend hours together on the porch watching sunsets and reminiscing. There was time for good byes for all of the friends and grandchildren. Although I have grown to hate the word closure, watching the cancer take my father slowly, allowed me to see and experience tiny pieces of closure each and every day. With mom it was the exact opposite. Each day was grabbed on to, held tight, never let go, lest the memory of that one sentence, one smile, and one conversation fade between us never to appear again. And then she was gone, first heart, soul and mind, later her physical being. After dozens and dozens of trips up and down the highway, thousands of miles on the car, too much money and cost to even count, too much heartache, it was over.

For the first time in my life, I did not want to be in charge of anything. My siblings handled all services, arrangements and decisions. I truly did not care. Worn out, spent, and hurt, I suddenly felt like an old orphan, now the oldest living generation. Grandparents gone, parents gone, aunts and uncles gone. My siblings and I advanced to the head of our family class. The oldest living generation and I did not like it.

I now wonder all of the time, what she knew, what and if she thought. How did she feel after she lost words. Did she know we helped her? Did she ever try to smile? Did she know we loved her?

Buster's Journey

Over the years I have always kept a journal. Not that I have an exciting life, just something I always enjoyed doing. During my husband's illness, I found that my journal was a release of emotions. After his death, it is a record of the life of two people and their struggle with dementia. Using quotes from my journal I will try to tell our story.

January 1999- He gets so confused. It really worries me. If he continues to get worse, how am I going to take care of him.

April 1999- Our doctor is so concerned with Buster's confusion. He has ordered more tests, an MRI and EEG. The diagnosis is small strokes called TIA's but not Alzheimer's at this time. I really have to watch him because it doesn't take much to confuse him.

June 2000- We went to Alabama to visit. During our time there I realized that Buster was worse than I thought. I decided to quit work to be home with him. That was a hard decision but my husband comes first. After 10 years working with the same company I walked away.

August 2000- Now that I am with Buster all the time I can see how really bad off he is. He isn't changing his clothes regularly and not bathing good.

September 2000- Doctor made Buster quit driving. That was hard because he didn't want to stop. We had a really bad fight over that but he gave me his license. A weight was removed from my shoulders.

February 2001- He is continuing to go down hill. He has now been diagnosed with Alzheimer's. He is very childlike. His communication skills are slowly going away.

July 2001- We went home to Alabama. Buster wanted to go back to his home at Union Hill. He wanted to see it all again before he forgets. He didn't do well. Each day he got more confused. He has gotten to where he has trouble getting his food onto his spoon to feed himself.

September 2001- Sometimes I get so upset. I try to be gentle and easy with him, but patience is a hard strive for me.

Buster got lost between bed and bathroom about 6:30 a.m. When I got up at 7:30 he was dressed. I asked him why he was up so early. He told me he got lost and this scared me. He seems to be loosing himself faster than I am ready for.

Getting close to 2002- Beginning of New Year. Lord be with us and Bless us.

February 2002- He seems to be doing okay but I can see a slow spiral down. He just gets duller and duller as time goes on. He sits out front a lot. He says its hot when it is 55 degrees just because the sun is shining. I am afraid he will chill.

March 2002- Buster has been more confused early mornings and late evenings. He sleeps so much. He is losing weight. In two weeks he has lost six pounds.

June 22nd, 2002- Buster had a stroke today. I had gone to get burgers for supper. When I got back he was really confused and anxious. I sure hope not much damage has been done. He ate his burger like he was starved so maybe not too bad.

June 25th, 2002- Buster's speech is worse. He gets some words messed up. He is moving slower and more stooped. We talked about if I leave him and come back and if he is sick again that he will go to day care from then on.

July 2002- Doctor put Buster on Depakote for the mood swings. He has been having temper tantrums. Buster seems to be getting worse each day. He has no concept of time. He will interrupt me notmatter what I am doing. He can hardly speak at all and his speech is very slurred.

August 8th, 2002- Buster can no longer be left alone. He gets lost in our house and our yard.

August 20th, 2002- I am so hurt over Buster's condition getting worse. It is getting more difficult to take care of him. He is getting clumsier and can not speak hardly at all. I know each day we are getting closer to him going into a nursing facility.

September 1st, 2002- He wet all over the floor and in his clothes twice. After washing all the towels and stripping the bed he did it all over again.

September 9th, 2002- Buster has fallen several times over the past few weeks. I have to get the neighbors to help me get him up. He wets the bed every night. I will have to put him in adult pull-ups. I have to take him to the bathroom now. He misses the seat when he goes to sit down if I do not guide him. I have had no more than three hours of straight sleep in a month. I get up with him at least four times a night to go to the bathroom. He wants so badly to care of himself.

October 6th, 2002- Sometimes he can't use his legs. It's so hard to hold him while I dress him. I have to get behind him to walk him from room to room.

October 12th, 2002- Not able to walk till late morning and by late afternoon not able to walk again. I told him I was calling the VA. I can't take care of him anymore. I can't lift and carry him. I am just worn out and beginning to break down. We both cried. I think he understands. This is so hard. I love him so and feel like I am letting him down.

October 16th, 2002-Admitted Buster to a living center with a special unit for dementia patients. He seems to understand but, of course, he doesn't want to stay. He had rather be at home and I would rather he were there too!

I sure hope this gets easier because right now I feel awful. I have let him down and feel so guilty. I was supposed to be able to take care of him. This is just all wrong.

My beloved husband passed away in his sleep on November 21st, 2002 at the age of 58. Our life together was good but the ending was so sad. Dementia takes away the dignity of the person and leaves life long doubt for the caregiver.

Granny

Granny was an awe inspiring woman. She was a strong Christian and lived a modest and very giving lifestyle until Alzheimer's Disease came into her life. At the time of her diagnosis, there was not a lot of information available, so we, as her family, kind of played hit and miss in the dark with ways to deal with her declining mental and physical health.

There were little things that we noticed off and on for several years, but we were all in denial. We can even look back to 1986 when my PaPa died, and remember things just prior to and just after his death, that pointed to Alzheimer's. It started with little things like leaving an open jar of mayonnaise out on the kitchen table, misplacing a pair of scissors, forgetting to take a bath or change clothes after an incontinent episode. It was frustrating dealing with her change in mental status. We all fought and argued with her about things that, really, there was no point in arguing over. We didn't know it at the time, but that only made her worse. We learned new things and ways of dealing with the frequent episodes after Mother joined an Alzheimer's support group. We had always been trained to reorient to person, place and time. With Alzheimer's, that can make a person affected by the disease, combatative and angry. Their reactions to different situations vary from person to person and from event to event.

After Granny took 6 hours to arrive at my Mother's home, a trip that normally only took 2 hours to drive, Mother took Granny's keys to her truck and made her move in with her and my brothers. Granny had evidently gotten off of IH10 to get something to drink and when she got back on the highway she was going West in the East bound lane of traffic. I don't know how she made it all the way to Van Horn in that lane but she did. My family went out looking for her and found her driving into oncoming traffic. For her safety and the safety of others it was best to take that action. Granny accused us of keeping her captive and frequently stole keys to the vehicles and tried to leave in them.

At first she was alright alone at the house for a few hours, but eventually we had to make other arrangements. She was a cook and had worked in the same restaurant for 30+ years, so it was natural that she would want to cook at home. We would come in to flames jumping off the stove, pans and food burned to oblivion. She would put things on to cook and go sit down and forget about them. Granny swore she didn't put that food on to cook. My oldest brother quit his job to stay home and care for Granny. We also had a provider who came in and would bath her and do things for her for 4 hours a day, just to give my brother a little break.

Granny had been living with my mother for about 2 to 2 ½ years, when I took her to my home for 2 weeks, so that mother could take a break from the stress. My brother came with her, so that there would be someone with her when I was at work. Granny took my car and disappeared for several hours one day. We had no other source of transportation and therefore could not go out looking for her. She did return, although I don't know how she found my house. She said she had gone to visit my PaPa at the cemetery. We have no idea if that is where she went or not, it doesn't matter. We just knew we had to sleep with the keys in our pockets and someone had to have her in eyesight at all times. We as a family found humor in dealing with this disease. It wasn't funny nor is it funny, but it was either laugh or cry. Laughing made the days seem better somehow.

Alzheimer's is a sad and cruel disease. Not only did it ravage my Granny's mind and body, it ravaged my family. Granny got to a point where she didn't know anyone or anything, but we still knew and we still know. Her mental death came long before her actual physical death. It was a blessing for not only Granny but also for my family when she finally passed from this life. Her legacy of life, love, giving to others and happiness will reign for lifetimes to come. Those of us who are left behind to cherish her memory will forever be affected by the woman that she was and the woman that she has become in death. I felt as if I died a thousand times over in grieving for the loss of her long before she died. I stayed with her until she drew her final breath in this world and saw the beautiful look of peace that flooded her face at that very moment. I knew then that life goes on, but leaves us with memories to keep forever deep in our souls.

Momma Dye

My grandmother known lovingly by most of her family and close friends as Momma Dye lived out her life and faced dementia with the help of her daughter and some key others the best she could. It is difficult to be faced with the few memories I have and the realization that I was not one of the key family members that helped her through her last years. I am unsure of when the diagnosis occurred but I do remember some years before nursing home placement that my grandmother started having trouble paying her bills and keeping up with her check book. This was one of the first signs noticed. She also became extremely paranoid towards her son and daughter about her money. She believed that her money had been taken by her kids. My Aunt lived on the same land with her and when her and her husband decided to build elsewhere they built a small one bedroom home for her on their new land. My aunt did everything she could to keep her safe, secure and well loved for as long as she could with the help of her children and grandchildren. The day finally did come where the decision was made to move her into a nursing home. Grandma stayed there until her death a few years later. She experienced all the stages of dementia. Her last days were spent bedridden, unable to eat or drink. The saddest part of it all is that I along with my dad had trouble understanding the disease process. Dad and I visited rarely. I even worked in her nursing home as a social worker and had trouble visiting. I did not know what to say. It made me uncomfortable when she thought I was my mom who had recently passed away. It was frustrating to carry on a conversation. Sometimes when I would visit she would be packing her things to go home and she would become anger and I did not know what to do. I thought I was making her angry. Unfortunately, the nursing home where my grandmother lived did not have much to offer at the time in regards to dementia education. Also keep in mind I was one of the social worker's where she lived! I felt so much anger, frustration, denial and confusion that is was easier to not visit. How unfair this was to my grandmother, Aunt and me! My aunt bore the responsibility of my grandmother's care with little help. Many years later looking back on that time I regret not understanding my feelings and realizing that it was normal. Everything I was experiencing was normal! Still working in the healthcare field with Alzheimer's almost 6 years after my grandmother's death with so much more education under my belt in regards to the entire process I decided to write a book on Alzheimer's dementia to help others find their light in that darkened tunnel. My hope is that you each will find light in the tunnel before your loved one passes away. For me that light did not come until years later but I will continue to learn, educate, speak and pass on everything I can to others in my grandmother's memory! I hope you learn from "Alzheimer's Days Gone By. " I know my grandmother would be proud to know that she was part of the reason why I overcame my fear of writing as well as the fear of success or worse yet failure to pass this information on to each of you! Enjoy those moments when the light burns so bright that it brings tears to your eyes!

Bibliography

Troubled with: A website of focus on the family. http://www.troublewith. com

Alzheimer's disease: Unraveling the Mystery. National Institute on Aging. Power Point based on this book.

Alzheimer's is the death of the mind before the death of the body. www. efmoody.com/lonterm/alzheimers.html

www.gmhfonline.org/gmhf/consumer/factsheets/caring_alzheimers_ disease.html

Alzheimer's disease and related disorder's association, Inc, 1990, 1999.

Alzheimer's Association Campaign for Quality Residential Care. 2005.

Caregiver Stress. Alzheimer's disease and related disorder association, 1995. Reprint 2004.

Steps to Assisting with personal care. Alzheimer's disease and related disorder association, 1999. Reprint 2003.

Steps to Caring for a person with late-stage Alzheimer's disease. Alzheimer's disease and related disorder association, 2000. Reprint 2004.

Steps to Enhancing Communication. Alzheimer's disease and related disorder association, 1999. Reprint 2004.

Steps to planning activities. Alzheimer's disease and related disorder association, 1996. Reprint 2000.

Steps to understanding challenging behaviors. Alzheimer's

disease related disorder association, 1996. Reprint 2004.

Bertram, L, Tanzi, RE. The current status of Alzheimer's disease genetics: what do we tell the patients?
Pharmacological research: the official journal of the Italian Pharmacological Society. Oct 2004; 50(4): 385-396.

Willis, SL, Tennstedt, SL, Marsiske, M, et al. Long-term effects of cognitive training on everyday functional outcomes in older adults. JAMA. Dec 20 2006;296(23):2805-2814.

Algase DL, Beck C, Kolanowski A, et al. Need driven dementia-compromised behavior: An alternative view of disruptive behavior. American Journal of Alzheimer's Disease. 1996;11(November/December):10-18.

Levey A, Lah J, Goldstein F, Steenland K, Bliwise D. Mild cognitive impairment: an opportunity to identify patients at high risk for progression to Alzheimer's disease. Clinical Therapeutics. Jul 2006;28(7):991-1001.

Knopman DS. Current treatment of mild cognitive impairment and Alzheimer's disease. Curr Neurol Neurosci Rep. Sep 2006;6(5):365-371.

Mark Rushing, Alzcare Assisted Living

Faison ,Fairia, and Frank (1999)

www.about.com/Alzheimer's
Elder Options of Texas, www.elderoptionsoftexas.com/library

www.alzheimertoronto.org/ti_intimacySexuality.htm

Intimacy, Sexuality and Sexual Behavior in Dementia, McMaster University, Hamilton, Ontario.

Sexuality and the Alzheimer's Patient. E. Ballared and C. Poer, Duke University Press, 1993.

A Thousand Tomorrows: Intimacy, Sexuality and Alzheimer's Disease(videotape). Terra Nova Films 1995
Disability Online. Victoria Australia

www.nia.nih.gov/nia.nih.gov/Templates/ADEARCommon/ADEARCommanPage.as

www.ivoryhouse.net/stressquiz

About the Author

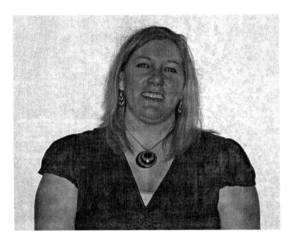

Deanna Lueckenotte received her formal education at University of Mary Hardin Baylor in Belton, TX and at University of North Texas in Denton, TX where she obtained her BA in Psychology. She then took 9 hours of her Master's at Baylor in Waco, TX. She has spent 8 years in long term care and during that time has received her Social Work License, Assisted Living certification and LNFA. She currently is an Executive Director at an Alzheimer's Assited Living in Southern Central Texas. During those 8 years she has been blessed by being able to work with people with Alzheimer's and their families. She also educates through the Greater Austin Alzheimer's chapter by educating on the basics of Alzheimer's for the 17 counties served. She has experienced personal loss from dementia. She loves to spend as much time as possible with her husband and son. They love to travel as much as possible. She recently added two new additions to their family, lab puppies! She likes to spend time with her extended family that also live in the Central Texas area.

If I am ever inflicted with this disease there is a good chance that I will go around singing or whistling to the tune of "Delta Dawn what's that flower you have on?" "Could it be a faded rose from days gone by?" The reason I would do this is because this song holds very strong childhood memories for me. My dad and I were always trying to sing or whistle this song. Please keep in mind that the person you are taking care of is living in their "Days Gone By."

To Book Deanna for a speaking engagement please email alzheimersdaysgoneby@live.com.

LaVergne, TN USA
21 August 2009
155547LV00001B/25/P

9 781438 967486